# Practice Management

## Keith Bolden

*General Practitioner and Senior Lecturer,*
*Department of General Practice, Postgraduate Medical School,*
*University of Exeter*

## Antony Lewis

*General Practitioner and Senior Lecturer,*
*Department of General Practice, Postgraduate Medical School,*
*University of Exeter*

## Brenda Sawyer

*Practice Manager and AHCPA Educational Co-ordinator*

OXFORD
BLACKWELL SCIENTIFIC PUBLICATIONS
LONDON EDINBURGH BOSTON
MELBOURNE PARIS BERLIN VIENNA

© 1992 K. J. Bolden, A. P. Lewis & Brenda
Sawyer

Blackwell Scientific Publications
Editorial Offices:
Osney Mead, Oxford OX2 0EL
25 John Street, London WC1N 2BL
23 Ainslie Place, Edinburgh EH3 6AJ
3 Cambridge Center, Cambridge,
   Massachusetts 02142, USA
54 University Street, Carlton,
   Victoria 3053, Australia

Other Editorial Offices:
Librairie Arnette SA
2, rue Casimir-Delavigne
75006 Paris
France

Blackwell Wissenschafts-Verlag
Meinekestrasse 4
D-1000 Berlin 15
Germany

Blackwell MZV
Feldgasse 13
A-1238 Wien
Austria

First published 1992

Set by DP Photosetting, Aylesbury, Bucks
Printed and bound in Great Britain by
Hartnolls, Bodmin, Cornwall

DISTRIBUTORS
Marston Book Services Ltd
PO Box 87
Oxford OX2 0DT
(*Orders:* Tel: 0865 791155
         Fax: 0865 791927
         Telex: 837515)

USA
Blackwell Scientific Publications, Inc.
3 Cambridge Center
Cambridge, MA 02142
(*Orders:* Tel: 800 759-6102
              617 225-0401)

Canada
Times Mirror Professional Publishing, Ltd
5240 Finch Avenue East
Scarborough, Ontario M1S 5A2
(*Orders:* Tel: 800 268-4178
              416 298-1588)

Australia
Blackwell Scientific Publications
(Australia) Pty Ltd
54 University Street,
Carlton, Victoria 3053
(*Orders:* Tel: 03 347-0300)

British Library
Cataloguing in Publication Data
Bolden, K. J. (Keith John)
   Practice Management.
   I. Title   II. Lewis, A. P.   III. Sawyer,
   Brenda
   362.172068

ISBN 0-632-03319-3

Library of Congress
Cataloging-in-Publication Data
Bolden, Keith J.
   Practice Management/
   K. J. Bolden, A. P. Lewis, Brenda Sawyer.
      p.   cm.
   Includes bibliographical references and
index.
   ISBN 0-632-03319-3
   1. Medicine--Practice.   I. Lewis, A.P.
II. Sawyer, Brenda.
III. Title.
   R728.B65   1992                91-45213
   610'.6--dc20                      CIP

# Contents

# Foreword

To be a manager in general practice in the Nineties is a challenge.

You need the same skills and qualities as the manager of any other business but with that extra special quality – the ability to care. To care passionately to manage and to lead change to the best of your ability. In addition you will make the most of every opportunity, constantly learning and developing your own skills and those of others to work together to improve the standard of practice management's contribution to patient care.

In the pages of this handbook the authors draw sensitively on their experience of both working in general practice and learning with teams of multi-disciplinary health care professionals. They provide the reader with encouragement, inspiration and motivation to look ahead. The scene is set against the background to the career of the general practice manager, where managers are today and, more importantly, where they are going. It is here the practical and realistic approach shines through this book. There are readable references and a real feeling of a wealth of opportunities for practice managers with new solutions to old problems.

A career in general practice management is an opportunity not to be missed and one, I am proud to say, this handbook supports.

*Sandra E. A. Gower*
*Practice Development Manager*
*Bennetts End Surgery, Hertfordshire*

*Past Chairman AHCPA*

# Chapter 1

# History and Development of General Practice

The word manager first appeared in a dictionary in 1588 but although the history of the general medical practitioner goes back for centuries that of the practice manager is relatively recent. The position of practice manager became established in the 1960s and their number has grown rapidly in recent years. A brief look at the developments in primary health care this century shows why this has come about.

By the end of this chapter you should:

1 Be aware of the development of the health care system in the UK.
2 Be able to appreciate the place of general practice within this system.
3 Understand how major policy documents affect the development of primary care.

## THE NATIONAL HEALTH SERVICE

### The National Health Insurance Act of 1911

The introduction by David Lloyd George (then a minister in the Liberal government) of the National Health Insurance Act of 1911 was the first step towards the provision of free health care, but only for a proportion of the population. It initiated registration with a general practitioner, insurance for working men earning less than £250 per year and provided financially for some of their treatment. It made no provision for their dependents who remained private patients. Workers, their employers and the Treasury contributed in differing proportions. In the case of illness, doctors who were participating in this 'panel' system gave medical attention free, and there was a weekly sickness benefit. Secondary care, dental and ophthalmic care were not covered.

Hospital doctors were regarded as the leaders of the medical profession but this Act was instrumental in establishing the concept of primary care, and the family doctor as its leader. Consultants were still dependent upon general practitioners for the referral of patients. The Act introduced a degree of state control, although this was perhaps balanced by increased financial security. Panel doctors still retained the right to private patients.

During the ensuing years, the general practitioner worked from home, 7 days a week and was available 24 hours a day. It was essentially a 'cottage industry' where the doctor's work was supported by his wife and family (there were then few women doctors). She often acted as the practice receptionist and it could be construed that the doctor's wife was the first 'practice manager'. Extra help was sometimes employed, usually in the person of a dispenser. In the first half of the century district nurses worked independently of general practitioners and there was little encouragement for collaboration. The nurses were then employed by the local authorities.

**The National Health Service Act of 1946**

In the 1920s and 1930s, as a result of the depression and with unrest amongst the working population, there was a growing movement for a more comprehensive medical service. Although plans were put forward by the Government and the British Medical Association, these were interrupted by the Second World War. However, during this interruption, William Beveridge in 1942 produced his seminal report. This advocated a Welfare State with the National Health Service (NHS) as its pivotal point for health care. The Labour Party campaigned for, and won, the first election after the war, with plans based on this report.

The National Health Service Act was passed in 1946. This gave all the population free access to general medical services. It continued and developed the capitation basis for remuneration and within each district the Executive Council became the administration body. The higher capitation fees gave increased remuneration, but did not encourage the practice of better medicine, the employment of support staff or working from adequate premises, as doctors were paid irrespective of the standard of their general medical services.

Conversely those doctors who did practise good medicine, employ appropriate staff and improve their premises were penalized financially. The receipt of regular quarterly remuneration relieved general practitioners of the necessity of charging and collecting private fees, although they were still allowed to have private patients. No longer could they sell the goodwill in their practices. There were still very few employed staff, as practices continued to be largely home based.

Hospitals were nationalized. Although the power gap between hospital doctors and general practitioners was narrowed a little there was dissatisfaction amongst general medical practitioners who felt isolated. They had few incentives to practise better medicine, no postgraduate education and no career structure. In contrast, those practising medicine in hospital were better rewarded, and were able to work with the advantages of direct access to pathology and X-ray services, which were not available to general practitioners except via consultants.

## The Royal College of General Practitioners

There were several reports produced during this time which highlighted the poor standard of practice. The Memorandum and Articles of Association of the College of General Practitioners were drawn up in November 1952. The foundation of this College enhanced the status of the general practitioner and when Prince Philip became Royal Patron in 1967 the name changed to include the word 'Royal'. The Royal Charter was granted on 23 October 1972. There were 1000 Foundation Members, but membership grew to nearly 17 000 in 1990 with 33 faculties. Prestigious premises at 14 Princes Gate were purchased in 1962.

The first university Department of General Practice was formed in Edinburgh in the 1960s. General practice was beginning to be included in the medical schools' curriculum and gave a basis for development of research in general practice. However, from the mid 1950s to the mid 1960s there was a decline in those entering general practice. It was seen as the place where 'failed' hospital doctors came to rest. Lord Moran's remark that general practice was for those who fell off the career ladder only served to confirm this opinion. The problem was exacerbated by the drain on the medical population which occurred with mass emigration to some Commonwealth countries in the early 1960s.

## Charter for the Family Doctor Service of 1966

Unrest in the medical profession in the 1960s about pay and conditions led to a threat by the profession to withdraw its services. The British Medical Association produced proposals for improvements and subsequent negotiations with the government led to a contract with better conditions, but it did not satisfy all the requirements.

A basic practice allowance was paid in full for those doctors who had at least 1000 patients, and *pro rata* payments to those with less patients. Additional payments were made for patients in excess of 1000 and capitation fees continued to be paid on top of this for general medical services. As an incentive to improve practice, item of service fees were introduced, for cervical cytology, immunizations, vaccinations, maternity and emergency work. Out-of-hours visits between 11 pm and 7 am were additionally remunerated.

It was recognized that doctors should have longer holidays and their working week be shortened. A condition was that they ensured that arrangements for the care of patients were made in their absence. They remained legally responsible for the provision of general medical services *in absentia*. One way of achieving these aims, and meeting the condition, was for doctors to form groups and this was encouraged by the payment of a group practice allowance. Many doctors formed partnerships (although this was not a requirement for payment of the allowance) and group practices enabled not only the sharing of work, in and out of hours, but also the sharing of expenses for premises, staff and equipment.

General practitioners cherish greatly their independent contractor status, which allows them the freedom to work independently making their own clinical judgements, and running their practice as they see fit.

Another provision was for payment of a postgraduate training allowance for the attendance at a required number of postgraduate training sessions. Further educational development was also supported by a requirement that each medical school set up a Department of General Practice. Financial provisions were made for the extension, modification or refurbishment of existing premises, or for the purchase of purpose-built premises or premises which could be substantially improved and this was facilitated by the formation of the General Practice Finance Corporation. Additional payments were to be made for the employment of ancillary staff.

Although doctors were encouraged by the new financial incentives to employ staff, reports showed that the numbers grew only slowly. Ann Cartwright's survey in 1967 indicated that only one-quarter of doctors employed any staff. However, 13 years later another report (Cartwright & Anderson 1981) found only 1% without either a secretary or a receptionist.

In the early 1960s health visitors were attached to some general practices and were followed by district nurses on an experimental basis. It was not until the Health Service and Public Health Act of 1968 that district nurses became officially attached to practices, rather than working on a geographical basis. A few doctors already directly employed practice nurses but from the early 1970s the numbers increased rapidly.

**Staff Associations**

There are two national associations which cater for general practice administrative and managerial staff.

In 1964 the Association of Medical Secretaries was founded. This latter expanded to include receptionists and practice administrators, and changed its name to the Association of Medical Secretaries, Practice Administrators and Receptionists (AMSPAR). Courses for these practice staff are organized through colleges of further education.

The Association of Health Centre and Practice Administrators (AHCPA) was formed by a group of health centre and practice administrators in 1975. It quickly grew and now embraces those responsible (together with their deputies) for the administration and management of practices. It is the leading national association which specializes in support and training for practice managers and this support is provided through a large branch network, and a regionally based training programme. Helpful packs on a variety of practice management related subjects are available.

The provision of health centres by local authorities was encouraged by the Government. The idea of health centres was not new and was mentioned in the Dawson Report of 1920. In the period from 1967 to 1981, 241 new health centres were built and by 1977 there were 842 in use in the United Kingdom. Doctors were encouraged to work in groups, not necessarily of the same partnership, by the payment of a group practice allowance. This was particularly useful for single handed general practitioners who could then take part in an out of hours duty rota but still qualify for the allowance because they worked in a group in this respect. However, many formed partnerships. These larger groups needed more organization and management which increased to the need for someone to carry out these roles other than the general practitioners.

**Vocational Training Act of 1977**

This act made vocational training mandatory from 1981. However, there had been trainees in general practice before this time. An early experiment in the 1960s was funded by the Nuffield Foundation and by the early 1970s vocational training had sprung up all over the country, funded by the government. The new act formalized this training and trainees were now required to work in rotation in selected specialities within hospital for a period of 2 years. A further year in general practice, if completed satisfactorily, led to a certificate of competence which permitted them to become principals.

During the 1980s there were a number of important reports:

1982    The Binder Hamlyn Report contained the potential for cost limiting in general practice.

1983    The Griffiths Report brought general management to hospitals and the community services.

1985    The Royal College of General Practitioners policy statement on quality.

1986    'Neighbourhood Nursing' – Julia Cumberledge's report called for more control, with nursing managers and locality management. She raised queries about the attachment of nurses to surgeries, favouring locality management.

1986    The Green Paper 'Primary Health Care: an Agenda for Discussion' mentioned a good practice allowance. It was clearly calling for the profession to look to put its house in order.

1987    'Promoting Better Health' gave Family Practitioner Committees (FPCs) a clear managerial role. This is the first time that managing general practice is mentioned.

1989    The White Paper 'Working for Patients' introduced general management into FPCs. Former FPC administrators had to apply for their jobs.

## General Practice in the National Health Service: The 1990 Contract

The contract which came into force on 1 April 1990 introduced new requirements for the provision of general medical services. One of these concerned the availability of doctors for patients. Doctors now had to spread their surgeries over 5 days a week, unless they were exempted for 1 day because they were undertaking other health-related work. They were required to be available for 26 hours a week solely for consultations in the practice over 42 weeks of the year. Visiting and administrative work was extra.

The 1990 contract made it easier for patients to change doctor by removing the requirement for them to obtain consent from their present GP or to notify their FPC.

The production of practice leaflets for patients and an annual report to the FPC became mandatory.

## The National Health Service and Community Care Act of 1990

The Green Paper 'Primary Health Care: an Agenda for Discussion' (1986) and the White Paper 'Working for Patients' (1989) formed the basis for the above act. The objectives of the Act were: better value for money; better patient choice; and better quality of service.

Family Practitioner Committees were to be known as Family Health Service Authorities (FHSAs). The new financial framework altered the flow of funds. Money went from the Department of Health to the regions, and thence to the newly named FHSAs, districts and general practice fund holders (GPFH). Money for non-fund holders came via the FHSA. Previously funds for the FPCs (and onwards to all general practitioners) had come directly from the Department of Health.

This act separated purchasers from providers and created GPFHs and hospital trusts. The advantage for NHS trust status was seen as giving more freedom to respond to the needs of patients by identifying with the local community. It would also give greater financial flexibility, and would enable the provision of a better quality of service to patients. The main disadvantages are the lack of consensus between main political parties on the issue and the suspicion of some NHS professional bodies and trade unions about trusts.

Section 60 of the act provided for the removal (with limited exceptions) from 1 April 1991 of the remaining Crown immunities enjoyed by the NHS.

The implementation of the new contract of 1990 brought changes to those involved in managing practices. Not only was there an increase in workload for all the practice team, but also the need for new skills. Managers were concerned with the complexities of the management of change. For some, those working in practices which were to become fund holders, there were two major changes within 12 months. Not only were business plans, annual reports and practice leaflets to be produced, but also there was a mandatory requirement for staff to be properly qualified and trained and for the setting up of health promotion clinics. There was a need for greater financial awareness with targets to be reached, and the cash limiting of reimbursement for staff.

Many doctors who had been previously undertaking administrative and managerial duties within their practices found that with the extra workload, they had to delegate to their existing manager, or to employ a manager. Many managers welcomed the new challenge. A large number had started in practice as a receptionist or secretary and been promoted to a managerial position. A survey of the members of AHCPA in 1991 showed that 49% of the 155 respondents were promoted from within, 71% of the promotions to manager taking place in the 1980s. However, some were happier to remain in their current role, and other people were employed to take on other managerial functions required for, say, fund holding.

Twenty per cent of the survey were fund holding in the first wave, or anticipated fund holding in the second wave. It was interesting that only 6% commenced work in general practice in the 1960s, and 33% in the 1970s, but during the 1980s it rose to 51%. The remaining started in 1990. The implications for general practice in relation to fund holding are explored later in this book. Fund holding commenced on 1 April 1991 for those practices in the first wave.

The role of the practice manager has always been challenging but never more so than in the face of the rapid changes occurring in the NHS at present. The authors hope that the rest of this book will give managers ideas and support to meet these challenges. Primary care may well look completely different in the next decade and practice managers will have to keep abreast of developments.

## FURTHER READING

Cartwright A. and Anderson R. (1981) *General Practice Revisited*. Tavistock, London.
*Evidence to the Royal Commission on the NHS.* Policy Statement 1. RCGP, November 1985.
*Quality in General Practice.* Policy Statement 2. RCGP, November 1985.
*Neighbourhood Nursing – A Focus for Care.* Report of the Community Nursing Review, HMSO, 1986.
Sawyer B. (1989) *The Professional Development of Practice Managers.* The RCGP Members' Reference Book, Sabrecrown, London.
*Working for Patients.* HMSO, 1989.

Further information can be obtained from:
The Secretary, AMSPAR, Tavistock House North, Tavistock Square, London.
The Membership Secretary, AHCPA, c/o 14 Princes Gate, Hyde Park, London SW7 1PU.

# Chapter 2

# The Role of the Practice Manager

Many practice managers are taking on a leadership role in general practice having entered the practice in other roles, such as receptionists, secretaries or nurses. They have grown with the developments in general medical practice, acquiring the new skills and knowledge needed to cope with the changing demands of this work. Their job descriptions have altered considerably over the years, as they have taken on greater responsibilities. Some were promoted to practice manager within their practice and others moved practice to take on the role.

Recently, with the increased demands of the new contract and fund holding, people with management and financial skills have been recruited from outside general practice. A survey in 1991 of AHCPA members showed that of the 6% who had started work in general practice in the 1960s, only one was a practice manager. Of those that responded who were promoted to practice manager from within, 68% were promoted in the eighties. Thirty-six per cent of respondents previously worked in the NHS and 14% in banks.

This chapter explores the areas that can make up the role of a practice manager. These are likely to apply to all managers irrespective of the size or location of their practice. At the end of the chapter you should:

1 Be able to use a management model as a tool in identifying specific areas for which you are responsible.
2 Have explored some ways of addressing these responsibilities.
3 Be aware of some of the rights and responsibilities of doctors.
4 Be aware of the rights of patients.
5 Understand how your role relates to others in the practice team.

There is no definitive job description for practice managers as the responsibilities and duties vary enormously from practice to practice. Some duties are relevant to the size and situation of a practice; the number of partners, the size of the list of patients, whether or not the situation is rural or inner city, if it is a dispensing practice. In some partnerships a doctor, or doctors, likes to play an active part in managing the practice, whereas at the other extreme there are doctors who include the practice manager in a partner role, with equal voting rights, and expect the manager to take on the entire management of non-clinical matters. Therefore, rather than detailing a job description, it is perhaps more useful to explore a model which can be applied to all situations in general practice.

John Adair, in his series of books on leadership, suggests such a model of management which is easily adapted to the role of a practice manager. He represents the three main areas to be managed as circles (Figure 2.1), each equally important but overlapping one another in part.

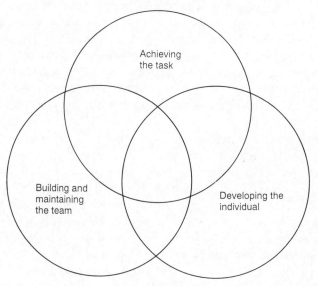

**Fig. 2.1**   Three main areas of management.

Each of the circles is equally important and certain areas overlap. For any manager, it is necessary to understand, support and develop those individuals for whom they are responsible. At the same time, it is important to ensure that they work effectively as a team, with good team spirit and interpersonal relationships. As individuals and team members, there is a task to be accomplished and a job to be done.

In general practice, this model can easily be applied to the reception area, the treatment room, the partnership team or, indeed, the entire primary health care team. Each individual is important and has differing needs, but these needs must be weighed against the fact that the team must be maintained. The manager needs to provide an optimum standard of service and care for patients and job satisfaction for staff. This model can be further developed and adapted to a management role in practice (Figure 2.2).

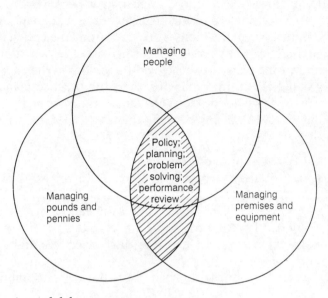

**Fig. 2.2**   A model for practice management.

As in the original model each of the circles has equal importance and in some areas are dependent upon, or reflect upon, one another. The central overlapping topics are the pivots around which the practice operates. To some extent, within each circle John Adair's original three circles could be placed, in as much as one should always be considering the individual, the team and the job to be done.

## POLICY MAKING

Each practice has its own philosophy, which in the past was largely formulated by the partners. This philosophy is not necessarily written down but can be deduced from the way the practice runs, the attitudes and relationships within and between members of teams, and the attitudes of patients and others involved in their care. However, practices are being encouraged to produce business plans and these usually include a mission statement, which encompasses the vision of the partnership.

## DECISION MAKING

Many managers now take part in the policy making and decision-taking in the practice, some having equal voting rights with partners on non-clinical matters. It is advisable to have a decision-taking policy. Although this may be unnecessary in single-handed practices, the larger the partnership the more important it becomes. This should perhaps place decisions to be made in categories, e.g. major, intermediate and minor. Major decisions would require all the voting members of the partnership team present, intermediate, a lesser number, and minor simply a majority vote. Placing the decisions in their appropriate category could fall to the senior partner, the practice manager, the chairperson of the meeting, or whoever seems appropriate.

John Adair (1985), in his book *Effective Decision-Making*, suggests a five-point plan:

*Define:* specify the aims and objectives.
*Collect information:* check facts, gather opinions, identify possible causes and time constraints, take into account other criteria.
*Develop options:* consider all possible courses of action.
*Evaluate and decide:* list the pros and cons, consider the consequences, measure against criteria, pilot, test against objectives and select the best.
*Implement:* brief everyone concerned, carry out decision, monitor and review.

## PRACTICE DOCUMENTS

The partnership agreement gives some details of how the partners wish to work together, share the workload and divide any profit.

The staff contracts and conditions of service (see Chapter 8) will reflect, in some part, the relationships between members of the staff and the partners, the benefits and the 'costs' of working for the practice.

Practices have different methods of recording protocols and procedures. Meetings are usually recorded in minutes, but 'standing orders' and methods of operating may be written in receptionists' handbooks, on a card index and such like.

### Business plan

A more recent policy document is the business plan. In compiling such a plan partnerships have found it necessary to work together to form a vision for their practice. It is necessary to look at where the practice is now, where it wants to be in the short and long term, and how it is going to get there.

This should commence with:

1   A mission statement – the vision of the aims and objectives that the practice would like to achieve.

2  A SWOT analysis
   (a)  Strengths – the strengths of the practice, in terms of resources and how they are used.
   (b)  Weaknesses – the weaknesses of the practice.
   (c)  Opportunities – the opportunities available to the practice.
   (d)  Threats – the threats to the practice (internal and external).

Although the practice manager may play a leading role in compiling the business plan, it is essential that all partners are involved as it is a statement of the partnership. This plan, together with the annual report, should be a well-used reference document for the practice.

## PLANNING

An important part of a manager's work is planning. An aid to this is another John Adair model, his planning cycle:

Define
Plan
Brief
Implement
Monitor support
Evaluate

and then back to re-define, starting the cycle again.

Before trying to formulate plans, it is essential to define what aims are to be achieved. Then, objectives can be set, and the steps to be taken discussed and planned. A timetable of actions to be taken will be helpful. Usually plans involve some form of change. Those individuals who will be affected and involved should be included as early as possible in the planning process. Briefing people is an important part of the planning cycle and this can be achieved either orally or in writing, or a combination of both. Once plans are implemented, it is necessary to monitor what is happening and to support those taking part. This monitoring and feedback will enable evaluation of the process, to ascertain whether or not the aims and objectives are being achieved. It might well be necessary to return to the beginning of the planning cycle to re-define the aims or objectives and start again.

One part a manager can play is in thorough research to find facts to help in the planning process. If a proposal is being made for change, to start something new, to purchase equipment, to employ a new member of staff, it is important to gather as much information as possible to help in making plans. If purchasing, obtain quotations and specifications from several sources, together with details of maintenance arrangements (if appropriate). If the proposal is to employ a new member of staff, it is necessary first to ensure that this would be more effective than to redeploy existing staff or the work. It is sometimes useful to produce a paper stating the facts, making suggestions, and to circulate this before the meeting.

## PROBLEM SOLVING

It is widely felt amongst practice managers that they need no more than 50% of their time to be allocated to routine jobs. The remaining 50% is then available to respond to the problems that arise in practice and much of this amounts to crisis management. Good time-management should be a skill that managers endeavour to learn. This is discussed in Chapter 12. In his book *Effective Teambuilding*, John Adair offers a useful framework for problem solving:

*Understanding the problem*

- Define the problem in your own words
- Decide what you are trying to do
- Identify important facts and factors

*Solving the problem*

- Check all main assumptions
- Ask questions
- List main obstacles
- Work backwards
- Look for a pattern
- List all possible solutions or ways
- Decide the criteria
- Narrow down to feasible solutions
- Select optimum one
- Agree implementation programme

*Evaluating the decision and implementing it*

- Be sure you used all the important information
- Check your proposed decisions from all angles
- Ensure the plan is realistic
- Review decision in light of experience

## PERFORMANCE REVIEW

### Medical audit

Medical audit became a requirement for general practitioners from April 1991. Medical Audit Advisory Groups (MAAGs) were set up by

FHSAs. Each group consists of general practitioners and other doctors experienced in audit. The aim is to maintain and improve the quality of care. The framework requires the committees to report regularly to FHSAs. A booklet *The Practice Audit Plan* by Richard Baker and Paul Presley explains in detail the reasons for medical audit, a practice audit plan, methods of collecting information and review. They state that the three main principles for a successful audit plan are that it should be:

1  Worker-centred.
2  Practice-based.
3  Problem-solving.

They describe a fundamental tool, the audit cycle. This consists of three basic steps:

1  To state what should be happening in any particular area to be audited.
2  To investigate exactly what is happening.
3  To discuss and plan how change can be introduced to satisfy the first statement.

Perhaps an additional step should be to assess how effective the change has been. All members of the team can be involved and it is one way of motivating people to take responsibility for what they are doing and the way they are doing it. Suggestions for audit can come from any member of the team. The first thought when mentioning medical audit may be that this should not involve practice managers. However, usually there are supporting administrative systems needed for the collection and collation of data, and non-medical members of the team may well be involved in this.

General practitioners are having to become more accountable and there is a growing awareness of the demand for a high quality of care. Audit enables the practice to examine where it is now, so that it can decide what it hopes to achieve and what it has to do to reach its goal. *Making Sense of Audit* (Irvine & Irvine 1991) helps unravel this process and concentrates on 'how to do it'.

Chapter 14 deals with audit in more detail.

## Appraisal

The performance of the team needs to be regularly reviewed. There are many methods of appraisal; staff, peer and self-appraisal being the best known. Each of these should involve examining the past and current performance, looking at strengths and weaknesses, and at positive plans of action to improve performance.

The practice manager has an important part to play in staff appraisal. It is essential that those being appraised are fully aware of what this means and of the aims of the exercise. A questionnaire for the appraisee to complete is a useful tool in facilitating the appraisal. This should explore how the appraisee perceives their personal strengths and weaknesses, what they feel could be done to help them to do their job better, and what they feel they need in the way of support and training to extend their skills. The answers can then be compared with the manager's view and during the interview differences in perception can be explored and positive action planned for the resolution of any problems and for the development of the member of staff.

The emphasis is on positive evaluation and positive action. Both parties should agree and sign the findings of the appraisal which should incorporate personal objectives and plans for the following period, usually a year. However, interim monitoring and support should be given.

Apart from individual performance review, there is a need to review the performance of the practice as a whole. The annual report is one way of accomplishing this and is now a requirement of FHSAs.

## PREMISES AND EQUIPMENT

The well-being of people who work in, and who visit, the practice can be affected by the state of the premises. In some deprived, inner-city areas it is difficult to maintain attractive buildings, inside or outside. Other areas are more fortunate, and with little vandalism and less wear and tear they are able to provide welcoming premises. Some practices have patient participation groups which help provide equipment, skills or funds for projects to improve their surgeries. Chapter 4 goes into detail about the management of premises and equipment.

## PEOPLE

When thinking of managing people it is usually the directly employed staff that come to mind first. A great deal of a manager's time is involved in the recruitment, selection, induction, supporting, training, motivating and appraising of staff. Detailed information about employment can be found in Chapter 8, and on relationships with other members of the primary health care team in Chapters 3 and 13.

The relationship between doctors and their managers has undergone great change recently. With the fresh requirements, and the increase in workload, generated by the 1990 contract, doctors look more and more to managers to share, or take over, the management workload. For those practices who were in the first wave of fund holding, one of the criteria for acceptance was that they were effectively managed. The general principles of management are discussed in detail in Chapter 12 but the following points are worth mentioning here.

## Communication

One of the main functions of a manager is that of communicator. It is essential that everyone knows what is expected of them and of others in the team.

### Internal

Some simple methods of communication are:

1  A white board in reception, visible to the team, but not to patients, on which any messages, or notices can be written. The use of different coloured pens can reinforce and attract attention.
2  A communications book, kept in reception where any member of the team can write messages for receptionists who sign when they have read each message. This is useful where there are part-time staff, as this ensures that everyone has the opportunity of keeping in touch.
3  Books for other members of the team, such as district nurses and health visitors, where messages are left for them to collect. These messages will come from various sources; patients, general practitioners, hospitals, social services, to name only a few.
4  Memoranda between members of the team.
5  Practice protocols and handbooks kept in appropriate accessible places, such as reception, office, treatment room or library.
6  Briefing sessions (say, 2 minutes each morning before surgery starts) making a statement about important issues of the day (e.g. a member of staff is off sick and work is being redistributed), a certain doctor needs to leave early and no extra patients can be seen, or to remember that there is a staff meeting that evening.
7  Messages flashed on VDUs where there is a networked computer system that has this facility.

### Meetings

A more complicated method of communication is through meetings. Managers are usually responsible for the convening and setting up of practice meetings. These can take various forms, formal or informal, in practice and externally, day-time and evenings or weekends, between members of the in-house teams or with others, such as patients or external people or organizations.

Within the team the composition of meetings can fall into many categories, but some common regular meetings may be between:

1   Doctors.
2   Doctors and practice manager.
3   Practice manager and staff.
4   Practice nurses.
5   Members from all groups within the primary health care team; doctors, nurses, health visitors, staff, chiropodists, speech therapists and so on.
6   Doctors and the directly employed staff team.

All expected participants at a meeting should be adequately briefed of the date, time, place and items to be considered. An agenda, with supporting documents where appropriate, circulated in advance can save time. People can then read beforehand what is to be discussed, research (if necessary), and get their thoughts together. The meeting will often run more smoothly if the expected time for discussion is placed against each item. Knowledge of the time-keeping of participants may lead to subjects of lesser importance being placed at the beginning and end, to cater for those who arrive late or leave early, thus keeping major decision taking in the middle, when all members are present. It is advisable to have a chairperson and someone taking minutes if a tape recorder is not being used. The roles of chairperson or note-taker may fall to the practice manager.

It is essential to record in the minutes decisions that are made and actions that are to be taken, by whom, and with any time restraints. One method of being able to check rapidly on past decisions is to extract all decisions from the minutes and place them under appropriate headings, with dates, in a reference book. For instance, the headings might include:

1   Finance.
2   Staff.
3   Trainee.
4   Premises and equipment.
5   Patients and services.
6   Health promotion.
7   Disease management.

It saves time spent trying to remember when a decision was taken and having to search through past minutes.

### External

It is essential that good communication is established between the practice and its patients. Patients should be aware of the services that are available from the practice, when they are available and how they may obtain them. Some methods used are:

1 Patient leaflets.
2 Posters.
3 Annual report (perhaps edited versions).
4 Patient participation groups.
5 Patients' newsletter.
6 By word of mouth from any member of the practice team.
7 Communications or complaints box in the waiting room.

## Rights and responsibilities

Perhaps the most important people whom managers must consider are the patients. They, too, have rights! Managers need to be aware of patients' rights, the main ones being:

1 To be on a general practitioner's list. They may choose a doctor as long as that doctor is willing to accept them. If they cannot find a doctor themselves the FHSA will allocate them to a list.
2 To see a general practitioner (not necessarily their own) during surgery hours. Where no appointment system exists, these hours should be clearly displayed on an external notice board. Where there is an appointments system, and a patient has not made an appointment, they should be given one at a later surgery as long as the wait will not be a risk to their health.
3 To be able to leave a message, 24 hours a day, 365 days a year.
4 To request a home visit, but the doctor has the right to decide whether or not it is necessary.
5 To obtain immediately necessary treatment from a general practitioner when away from home in cases of urgent need.
6 To change general practitioner. The FHSA must make sure the patient is not without a doctor.
7 To confidentiality. Doctors should not pass on information about patients except to other people involved in their treatment, and, in certain cases, to close relatives. For children under 16 years old parents or guardians have a right to information. However, if a doctor suspects that a child is being deliberately abused they may pass this information on to the local authority social services department or the NSPCC.

It is advisable that practice managers make themselves aware of the rights and responsibilities of doctors in the general practice setting. For instance, the issue of confidentiality mentioned above can affect all members of staff as well as doctors and there should be a practice policy on such procedures.

Another area to be addressed is that of drugs, in particular the safe and secure storage and logging of the use of, dangerous drugs. The Misuse of Drugs Act of 1971 details certain requirements relating to drugs and the *Practice Nurse Handbook* (Bolden & Takle 1989) gives advice on this subject). For instance, controlled substances must be kept in a locked cabinet or cupboard and a register kept on the premises. This register must record the date of purchase, the amount, batch numbers, and the supplier. Details of distribution, whether to a patient or for a doctor's bag, must also be recorded.

## CONCLUSION

The role of the practice manager has seen a major transformation since senior receptionists occasionally adopted the title of 'practice manager'. There is no doubt that this role will continue to expand rapidly as the decade progresses and the setting of primary care will continue to change. Practice managers have a very exciting and challenging time ahead.

## REFERENCES

Adair J. (1985) *Effective Decision Making*. Pan Books Ltd.
Blanchard K. & Johnson S. (1983) *The One Minute Manager*. Fontana Paperbacks.
Bolden K.J. & Takle B. (1989) *The Practice Nurse Handbook*, second edition. Blackwell Scientific Publications, Oxford.
Irvine D. & Irvine S. (editors) (1991) *Making Sense of Audit*. Radcliffe Medical Press.

## FURTHER READING

Irvine D.H. (1990) *Managing for Quality in General Practice*. King's Fund Institute, London.
Jones R.V.H., Bolden K.J., Pereira Gray D.J. & Hall M.S. (1985) *Running a Practice*, third edition. Croom Helm, London.
The National Consumer Council and the Association of Community Councils for England and Wales issue a leaflet *Patients' Rights: a summary of your rights and responsibilities in the NHS*, obtainable from the association at 30 Drayton Park, London N5 1PB. It is also printed in several languages other than English.
*Rights and Responsibilities of Doctors*, published by the BMA.

# Chapter 3

# The Primary Health Care Team

## INTRODUCTION AND OBJECTIVES

The concept of teamwork and some of the elements underlying its structure are discussed elsewhere in this book (Chapter 13). This chapter looks at personnel in the typical primary health care team, exploring their background, terms of service and future needs.

At the end of this chapter you should:

1 Understand the roles of individual disciplines within the team.
2 Understand their background.
3 Understand some aspects of a practice partnership.
4 Understand the terms of service of personnel in the primary health care team.
5 Understand the continuing needs of individual members of the team.

A primary health care team is a group of professionals working together for the social good of a group of clients. Usually the team consists of general practitioners, the manager and reception staff of the surgery or health centre, practice nurses, community nurses, midwives and health visitors. Other teams may include social workers, counsellors, physiotherapists, community psychiatric nurses and occasionally other specialist professionals (for example occupational therapists and marriage guidance counsellors).

## GENERAL PRACTITIONER

All patients are registered with a single doctor. The general practitioner (GP) is thus the common link in the primary health care team. The GP may regularly assume leadership of the team, but leadership may vary from situation to situation. For example, at times the health visitor may lead, as when child health development clinics are set up. Similarly, others may take the lead when their particular skills are called upon.

A vacancy may be created by the death or retirement of a practitioner. Any other vacancy cannot be filled without permission from the FHSA and Medical Practice Committee (MPC). The MPC is a committee based in London that must approve all new practice vacancies. Areas in the UK are designated as either open, restricted or closed. In open areas doctors can set up practice on their own with no established list of patients. Such areas are now rare, most being either restricted or closed.

GPs work in partnerships. Most have a partnership contract, though a surprising number still do not. Legally, even though a contract does not exist, partnership law applies where a group agree to work together sharing the profits and this constitutes a partnership. The content of a partnership agreement varies from group to group. Standard contract forms can be used but it is sensible to seek the advice of a solicitor, as amateur contracts may not be legally sound. An example of this is a clause restricting the ability of an outgoing practitioner to practice within a certain distance of the old practice and for a certain time. Courts of law now tend to take the view that it is unreasonable to restrict the ability of a person to earn a living by means of their vocation. The existing partners select a successful candidate from those who have applied for the job. This is discussed more fully in the chapter on teamwork.

Although all GPs are self-employed, many have extra employment outside the practice. Some are clinical assistants or hospital practitioners in the local hospital. Others have employment as doctor to a local industry; yet others are employed as school doctors. Such income may be taxed at source, but it should be possible for the practice accountant to negotiate for it to be paid untaxed, therefore conforming with most partnership agreements.

GPs have a legal contract with FHSAs to provide care 24 hours a day, 7 days a week and 52 weeks a year. The terms of this contract are laid out in detail in the terms and conditions of service (The Red Book), a copy of which is essential for any practice manager. The FHSA is responsible to the Regional Health Authority (RHA), a group of elected people whose chair is appointed by the Secretary of State for Health. Each RHA is in turn responsible to the Secretary of State. District Health Authorities have no control over FHSAs nor GPs, though FHSAs co-operate with them in planning the health needs of a community.

Trainees are employed by the trainer who receives reimbursement of the salary from the FHSA. The trainee's pay is subject to PAYE as is the pay of other staff members. The trainee will also receive an allowance for running a car but whether this is taxed at source or given as an expense to the trainee in return for motoring receipts is a debatable point and recommendations vary from tax office to tax office. It is advisable to discuss this issue with your accountant.

GPs are encouraged to participate in continuing education, more so since the introduction of the postgraduate education allowance (PGEA) in April 1990. This allowance is given to GPs if they have completed 5 days of training in the preceding year. This training must contain a blend of courses from three areas – health promotion, disease management and service management, and may take place in the practice or at a postgraduate centre. Recognition may also be obtained for distance learning courses and some personal studies. It is useful to obtain details of PGEA recognition of practice-based clinical meetings and personal study from the local regional adviser's office. Full details of the allowance are given in the Red Book.

## PRACTICE NURSE

The idea of having a nurse employed by the partnership and working mainly within the surgery premises developed rapidly during the 1970s. The practice nurse is responsible to the partners, the employers. This requires the partnership to be certain that the nurse is competent to undertake the tasks that are stipulated in the job description. Liability for error may rest with the partnership if this is not clarified. It is clearly important that the practice nurse is adequately insured. Royal College of Nursing indemnity is adequate for this, but the defence unions also provide special cover, details of which may be obtained on request.

In common with all employees, the practice nurse should have a contract with a detailed job description. The content will vary from practice to practice. All practice nurses provide basic nursing care, such as dressings and injections, and are usually involved in the taking of cervical smears. Many also provide health promotion clinics, such as weight, hypertension and asthma clinics. The decision on whether practice nurses should undertake duties at the reception desk is debatable. Issues such as these need to be clarified at the start of a practice nurse's term of service.

In many groups, the practice nurse is used by patients as the first contact with the team, particularly if they are uncertain whether to consult a doctor over a minor problem. The nurse can often reassure the patient about the problem but is unable to prescribe medication, though a particular course of treatment may be recommended. In the United States, the nurse practitioner is able to prescribe certain medications such as the oral contraceptive. It is possible that in the future practice nurses will move in this direction.

Within a detailed job description, it is advantageous for practice nurses to function as independent professionals. This allows them to organize their clinical and administrative work and ensures job satisfaction. Health promotion and screening clinics increase the importance of this independent role.

When calculating whether or not a practice can afford to employ a nurse, it is important to consider both the income a practice nurse generates as well as doctors' surgery time saved. Seventy per cent of the practice nurse's pay will probably be reimbursed by the FHSA but before appointing a new nurse, or considering upgrading the pay of an established nurse, it is important to verify with the FHSA that reimbursement will occur.

Many nurses will have had special training beyond basic nurse training. This may include training in clinical areas such as the management of asthma, or in specialized areas such as family planning. Further training for practice nurses is now available in many centres. There is no stipulated annual quota of training a nurse should undertake. Increasingly, practices are feeling that all staff members should undergo the same amount of training as the GPs in the team – that is a minimum of 30 hours per year. The amount of training and the duties carried out by the practice nurse help determine their level of pay, which needs to be agreed with the FHSA before the start of employment. Training needs are discussed further in Chapter 11.

## OFFICE STAFF

The needs of individual practices vary but many practices are now employing managers. The manager may have a deputy or administrative assistant to free time for planning and other key managerial matters. There are also others in the team, such as a senior receptionist, secretary and computer operator.

Smooth running of the GPs' surgery revolves around the office and its ability to process appointments, therefore, an efficient team of receptionists is vital. Whether full or part time staff are employed may have a historical basis in the practice. It is important to consider the merits and disadvantages of both forms of working before deciding whether or not to perpetuate the status quo. Whichever system a practice chooses, the manager must ensure that approval has been given by the FHSA for reimbursement for the receptionists' pay. FHSAs now require practices to give an estimate of staff changes, as well as reasons why the changes are necessary, in the forthcoming year in the annual report. Without this notice it seems unlikely that the FHSA will give approval for expensive changes in the practice staff arrangements.

FHSAs reimburse 70% of receptionists salary and levels of pay are usually linked to the Whitley scale. Practices are of course free to pay staff the salary they feel is appropriate, but FHSAs are very unlikely to reimburse salaries in excess of the appropriate grade on the Whitley scale. Many FHSAs expect all new staff to be placed on the lowest scale for their grade despite previous experience. Early negotiation with the FHSA over scales of salary for new staff is clearly important. It would be unwise to offer a potential recruit to the office staff a salary without having checked this with the FHSA.

Receptionists are pivotal to the successful functioning of the practice. Besides ensuring the smooth operation of the appointment system, they have to deal with anxious and distressed patients. They are often the butt of frustration and anger. They have to process repeat prescriptions, file the notes accurately and answer the telephone, deciding whether calls are urgent or not. It is a stressful job. Good managers monitor stress levels carefully, and have systems for defusing tense situations. Clear protocols for the different jobs help and other systems designed to praise good work and to monitor for errors are also useful.

New receptionists need training in the skills of their new post. This can either be provided 'in house', or courses are available in all centres provided by professional bodies such as AMSPAR or the local FHSA. Basic skills should be covered on these courses, but much of the receptionist's work is in dealing with distressed people, and interactional skills need to be taught. This area is probably best covered in the practice as a team, when not only new receptionists, but also the experienced, can learn together. Many teams hold study days or weekends when all members of the PHCT gather to explore topics relevant to all.

There is no statutory requirement for continuing training for office staff, but FHSAs require information of training that has been provided over the year, in the annual report, and notice of study leave must be given for FHSA approval for payment. It is possible that in the future, reimbursement for staff may bear some relation to the amount of training given. As with nursing staff, many practices feel that office staff should have the same amount of study leave as principals, that is 30 hours a year.

## COMMUNITY NURSES

Whereas practice nurses work mainly in the surgery, community nurses visit patients in their home. They have registered nursing qualifications as well as special experience and training in home nursing. They are responsible to the community nursing officer, and though they may work within the boundaries of one practice, may also share patients with other practices.

The role of the community nurse is to assess the needs of patients who are ill at home, providing such nursing care as is necessary. Without the help of the community nurse, it would be impossible to care for many sick people at home. The nursing care involved includes tasks such as bathing patients who are ill, but this more routine work is frequently delegated to a bath nurse. Similarly, many community nursing teams have auxiliaries working with them who may be delegated work by the nursing sister. Some but not all community nurses carry out work such as venepuncture or ear syringing; views on this differ from area to area and depend on direction from the nursing officer.

Community nurses are paid by the District Health Authority, who also provide funds for the equipment they need and are responsible for their further training. They require prescriptions for medications and dressings from GPs. As the organization of the community nurse's day is complex and includes travelling from patient to patient, it is helpful if such prescriptions are processed rapidly. Meetings with the GP to discuss particular patients' needs are also necessary, and a regular time when contact with the GP can be guaranteed is helpful.

Community psychiatric nurses (CPNs) are also employed by the health authority. Their role is to care for psychiatrically ill patients. Their aim is to help prevent admission to hospital, and to achieve this aim they need to liaise closely with other members of the PHCT. CPNs are registered nurses who have had specialized training in dealing with psychiatric problems. This enables them to undertake treatment as well as the assessment and monitoring of people with mental health problems. This treatment may include counselling or behaviour therapy. A similar role is performed by community nurses with a special training in working with people with a learning disability.

Midwives are nurses who have had specialist training in the delivery of babies and the care of pregnant women. Birth rates are such that it is likely that a midwife is attached to more than one PHCT. Employed by the health authority, the midwife has a similar position to that of the health visitor. Antenatal clinics, which take place in the practice, are usually shared between the GP and the midwife. Midwives are also involved with home deliveries, though these are now much less frequent. They may also attend the labour ward for the delivery of mothers who have been in their care during the antenatal period.

## HEALTH VISITORS

Health visitors are registered nurses who have had extra training in the problems of public health. This training gives them special skills in managing the problems of the very young, mothers and the elderly. Health visitors have a statutory duty to visit all newborn babies on or about the eleventh day of life. Clearly this brings them into contact with many vulnerable sections of society. They are thus important sources of support for the needy and deprived.

As with community nurses, health visitors are employed by the District Health Authority, who also provide funds for equipment. They are, however, attached to a particular group, and work closely with that team. They are responsible to the local nursing management team, but in practice are usually free to organize their work around the needs of the PHCT.

An important role of the health visitor is to organize developmental screening clinics for the under fives. In these clinics, babies and young children are monitored to confirm they have no physical abnormalities, as well as to confirm that their development is normal. GPs may be involved in these clinics as well. Since the introduction of the contract in 1990, GPs with recognized skills in child care are paid a fee for each child on their list under the age of five.

Immunization uptake is an important role for the health visitor. Advice is given to mothers on when each immunization is given. Some mothers have fears about immunizations, particularly that for whooping cough, and the health visitor can help allay anxieties. Now that practices are expected to reach 90% immunization rates before being paid, the role of the health visitor has taken on new financial implications for the partnership.

Some authorities employ health visitors with a special interest in the elderly and screening and visiting of the elderly enables this role to expand.

## OTHER ATTACHED PERSONNEL

The conditions of employment of the following personnel vary. They offer services that can augment the treatment delivered by the practice. As in all multidisciplinary work, communication networks are vital.

Increasingly, social workers are linking with PHCTs to the benefit of their clients. They have special skills in helping the underprivileged of society. They have many statutory duties, mainly related to children, but also with other vulnerable sections of society, such as those with mental illness. They are also involved with the homeless, the elderly and those who need the provision of extra care at home. They are employed by the local department of social services.

Counsellors are working more often within primary care. Psychologists and other trained counsellors provide a valuable service to patients who have personal or emotional problems. Marriage guidance counsellors may undertake sessional time within the practice building, as may other specialized counsellors such as those from CRUSE (supporting those who are bereaved).

There are nurses with very specific skills in helping people with particular problems. Examples of these include Macmillan and Marie Curie nurses, who have skills related to the care of the dying, diabetic liaison nurses, continence advisers and stoma care nurses.

Physiotherapists have found a role in some PHCTs. Their main responsibility is to care for acute injuries and other acute physical problems such as back problems. They have an important place in advising on the prevention of many physical problems such as back strain. Other professionals allied to medicine, such as occupational therapists do not yet seem to have an established role in the PHCT. With their special interest in rehabilitation and adjustment to chronic disability, either physical or psychological, their role can be expected to expand.

## CONCLUSION

With the changes in funding of general practice, and a greater freedom for PHCTs to decide how their funds should be spent, it is probable that PHCTs will have a wider range of professional representatives in them. This will particularly affect budget holding practices, who can expect to have a greater choice on how to spend their funds. It seems clear that with the justifiable increase in patient expectations, membership of the PHCT will expand, being complemented by more external resources.

# Chapter 4

# Premises and Equipment

General practitioners need adequate premises from which to provide services for their patients. The contents of this chapter should enable you to:

1  Discover how to plan for the acquisition of new, or modification of existing, practice premises.
2  Be conversant with laws relating to premises, including the Health and Safety at Work Act and Control of Substances Hazardous to Health regulations.
3  Keep relevant records relating to premises and equipment.
4  Ensure appropriate monitoring of the cleanliness and state of repair of buildings, fixtures and fittings, and of equipment.
5  Find out more details from relevant sources.

The 1966 Charter established arrangements for the reimbursement of rent for qualifying premises. General practitioners who own, or rent, a pre-existing building, used as practice premises, are reimbursed under a direct arrangement, dependent upon the market rent of the premises. However, in the case of separate, purpose-built premises, application for reimbursement should be based on the cost of the premises rather than on the market value.

## COST-RENT SCHEME

The cost-rent scheme enables general practitioners either to build completely new premises, or to purchase, lease or rent premises which require substantial modification, or to substantially modify existing practice premises.

### Where to find help if embarking upon a cost-rent scheme

*FHSA* – some have lists of suitable architects. Many employ specialist advisors or have staff acting as facilitators. They will advise on what may be acceptable, including siting, design and potential problems relating to access and services.

*'Red Book'* – The Statement of Fees and Allowances, para 51. Detailed information is available here, but is sometimes difficult to interpret. The sizes of rooms are laid down with the maximum costs that will be reimbursed and limitations on their use.

*Banks* – some banks have special medical managers who are able to advise on raising finance for practice premises.

*Local council* – for rules and regulations relating to planning permission, and building work.

*Accountant* – will advise on the financial aspects, in particular relating to the share each partner wishes to have in say, the purchasing of new premises. Those accountancy partnerships with specialist medical departments should be familiar with the Cost-Rent Scheme.

*Solicitor* – will carry out conveyancing on the purchasing of property and advise on legal implications, including any changes needed to the partnership agreement.

*Medical Architecture Research Unit* – has the latest information on research.

*Royal Institute of British Architects* – produces a booklet, *Architect's appointment – Small Works*.

*HMSO* – General Medical Practice Premises Health Building Note 4b, 1989.

It is also advisable to visit other purpose-built premises to obtain ideas, and learn of the experiences of colleagues.

## Procedure

At the outset, it is desirable to appoint one person (a GP or practice manager) as a project manager. This person will be the central contact, co-ordinate the project and liaise with all involved parties.

Once appropriate research has been carried out, a possible site selected and a project manager appointed, a suggested procedure is:

1  Contact the local FHSA, who will have people with experience in the development of surgeries and the cost-rent scheme.
2  Give in-depth consideration to the requirements of the practice in the planning of the new or modified premises: the number and position of consulting rooms, including one for a trainee if applicable; the placing and type of treatment room, administration office, reception and waiting area; accommodation for staff; the siting of computer, telephone and filing systems.
3  Submit an outline proposal to the FHSA with a rough estimate of timings. Although their approval may be forthcoming, there is no

guarantee at this stage that the money will be available.

4   Ensure that outline planning permission is available for the selected site and investigate in detail any restrictions associated with it. These may have a bearing when the district valuer carries out an assessment and makes recommendations to the FHSA.

5   Contact the expected source of funding for the project (e.g. bank, solicitor and accountant) and hold preliminary discussions. The accountant will advise on whether or not it will be possible to register for VAT during the building process. This will enable the practice to reclaim VAT on certain expenditure over a limited period of time.

6   Employ an architect, who will make a feasibility study and draw up outline plans of the buildings and rooms, together with a preliminary timetable. This architect will contact the local planning authority in order to seek the necessary statutory permissions and comply with local bye-laws. It is advisable to engage a quantity surveyor, either through the firm of architects, or perhaps recommended by the FHSA. Similarly, an independent surveyor will be needed during the project. The quantity surveyor will make an initial estimate of the costs of the project. It is preferable that the architect should be experienced in dealing with practice premises, as he, or she, should be aware of the latest rules and regulations (such as access for the disabled), and informed on issues associated with confidentiality within the building. The independent valuer will assess the completed value of the surgery and it is upon this assessment that a lender will base the viability and size of a loan. It therefore follows that a high estimate is advantageous.

7   Submit these plans to the FHSA supported by justification for application.

8   A written offer from the FHSA will confirm a preliminary assessment of reimbursement, the method for calculating this, and the dates acceptable for start and finish of the project. (NB If the building is not completed by the target finish date, the FHSA can withdraw their approval, and costs to date will not be reimbursed.)

9   The architect draws up the final plans (all changes at any time in the project must be notified to the FHSA for approval), which must be submitted to the local authority and to the FHSA.

10   Obtain final planning permission.

11   Research into suitable building companies should be carried out. Large companies often have high overheads, whereas small companies might not be able to cope with the size of the project. District Health Authorities usually have a list of approved

companies, which will have been financially vetted. Letters of invitation to tender are then sent to builders thought to be suitable, asking them if they would like to submit a tender. Go out to tender. These tenders should be based on exact specifications and should be a 'fixed-price', with contract variations only if the practice changes the requirements or for legislative changes. The local fire brigade are able to advise on the latest fire regulations.

12   It is usual for the architect to call for the three lowest tenderers to submit a copy of a priced bill of quantities for checking with the quantity surveyor. The tender should be accepted and a building contract signed. The architect will, in case of need, from now on act as an arbitrator between the practice and the builders.

13   Arrange appropriate insurance for the building site. Interim payment certificates, based on information from the builder and quantity surveyor, should be issued by the architect to the building contractor, who submits them to the practice for monthly payment.

14   Monitor the building programme and select fixtures, fittings, furnishings and equipment.

15   When the building is ready for occupation, a certificate of completion signed by the architect must be submitted to the FHSA, together with receipted accounts.

The cost-rent is payable only from the date that the premises become fully operational.

## REPAIR AND MAINTENANCE OF BUILDINGS AND EQUIPMENT

It is desirable to have presentable, well-maintained premises for patients to visit, and in which people can work. One way of effecting this and of containing costs is to monitor buildings regularly. Those working in District Health Authority owned premises will have a department, e.g. Works, Estates or Supplies Department, which responds to the need for maintenance, repair and renewal. However, it is still necessary for a manager, or administrator, responsible for the premises to identify the need. Sometimes a caretaker is employed to assist in this area. One method of managing this element is to have a regular monitoring check list for external and internal examination (Table 4.1).

The Estmancode, published in the 1970s by the Department of Health, gives guidelines which are used in the NHS. They divide maintenance work into four categories:

1   Planned preventive maintenance: regular scheduled servicing, for example the cleaning of gutters, the servicing of autoclaves.

**Table 4.1** Maintenance checklist.

|  | Condition | Action needed | Date reported | Date actioned |
| --- | --- | --- | --- | --- |
| *External* |  |  |  |  |
| Roof |  |  |  |  |
| Guttering/pipes |  |  |  |  |
| Drains |  |  |  |  |
| Windows |  |  |  |  |
| Doors |  |  |  |  |
| Brickwork |  |  |  |  |
| Signs |  |  |  |  |
| Lights |  |  |  |  |
| Grounds |  |  |  |  |
| *Internal* |  |  |  |  |
| Floors |  |  |  |  |
| Walls |  |  |  |  |
| Ceilings |  |  |  |  |
| Woodwork |  |  |  |  |
| Furnishings |  |  |  |  |
| Fittings |  |  |  |  |
| Furniture |  |  |  |  |
| Equipment |  |  |  |  |

2 Irregular maintenance: attend to slowly developing problems as required, for example repointing of brickwork.
3 Repair of breakdown or fault correction: for example radiator leaks, replacement light bulbs.
4 Small improvements/additions: for example fitments for new equipment.

During regular inspections, careful attention should be paid to health and safety conditions and safe practices. Trailing cables from equipment, receptionists using unsafe methods of climbing to reach medical records, and such like, are hazardous and need attention.

Useful tools in managing premises are log books. For example, in one a record is kept in date order of events relating to the building, requests for work to be carried out, dates of completion, by whom done and cost. It could also contain details of whom to contact with regard to plumbing, electrical work, gas, telephone, etc. In another, equipment is listed in alphabetical order with cost, date of purchase, identification details, details of vendor, guarantee or maintenance terms and cost of maintenance. Details of maintenance and repair are entered as they occur. For those who prefer to use the computer, there are databases available.

8

## HEALTH AND SAFETY AT WORK ACT 1974

The above Act was an enabling act which was in addition to other legislation such as the Factories Act and the Offices, Shops and Railway Premises Act. In some parts, it replaced these Acts, but many of the regulations of the old Acts remain current. There is continual amendment and it is wise to keep up to date with requirements. For instance, on 1 April 1991, crown immunity for those working in District Health Authority owned health centres ceased.

The aims of the act which directly affect practices are:

1  To ensure the health, safety and welfare of persons at work.
2  To protect people, in addition to employees, against risks to health and safety, arising out of or in connection with the activities of persons at work.
3  To control the keeping and use of explosive or highly flammable or otherwise dangerous substances, and generally preventing the unlawful acquisition, possession and use of such substances.

Regulations apply to all persons at work, with the exception of domestic servants in private households. Section 2 of the Act lays down the general duties of the employer, the first part, Section 2.1, stating:

> It shall be the duty of every employer to ensure, so far as is reasonably practicable, the health, safety and welfare at work of all his employees.

For practices, this means that equipment, machinery and systems of work must be as safe as possible, and with no risks to health. An example might be the handling and transport of blood samples or dangerous substances such as nitrous oxide.

The environment in which employees work must be safe and without risks to health. For directly employed staff, the Act also covers their welfare.

There is also a responsibility upon the practice for the protection of patients and other visitors to the surgery. Section 3.1 states:

> It shall be the duty of every employer to conduct his undertakings in such a way as to ensure, so far as is reasonably practicable, that persons not in his employment who may be affected thereby are not thereby exposed to risks to their health and safety.

Such good practices might be the strategic placing of 'Wet Floor' signs to ensure that patients do not slip when a floor has been washed, or ensuring a clear passage in the corridors, with no obstacles likely to cause an accident.

Health and Safety Inspectors have the right to enter premises at any reasonable time if they believe it is necessary under the terms of the Act. They have the power to examine or investigate, to take photographs and recordings, or to require a person to give information. They may be accompanied by any duly authorized person, but may be required to produce a copy of his instrument of appointment.

The inspector may take the following actions if the Act has been contravened:

1  Issue a prohibition notice (in an instance where there may be risk of serious personal injury).
2  Issue an improvement notice (this gives time for the fault to be remedied within a specified time).
3  Prosecute a person contravening the act.
4  Seize, render harmless or destroy anything which he considers might be the cause of imminent danger or which might cause serious injury to a person.

Free leaflets giving more information can be obtained from the local offices of the Health and Safety Executive.

## FIRE REGULATIONS

It is essential that everyone is aware of the procedure in case of fire. Even in the smallest organization, people should know what is expected of them. A fire procedure should be posted in an easily visible location (see Figure 4.1). This should detail who does what, and who goes where. Fire exits should be marked; fire doors kept closed. Each employee, as part of the induction training, should be informed of fire procedures, and anyone who is to spend time working in the building should be trained likewise.

When reporting a fire, there can sometimes be a tendency to forget the exact address and telephone number of the premises. Labels on each telephone terminal, giving these details can save time and possibly lives. The local fire brigade officers or, in some districts, the health authority fire officers give lectures and can arrange special fire drills.

## SECURITY

The local Police Crime Prevention Officers are able to give expert advice on the best precautions to be taken for safeguarding the security of practices. They will suggest measures that can be taken for external and internal security of the buildings; procedures for protecting the personal property of staff, drugs, practice equipment, and prescriptions; and ways of dealing with vandals and intruders.

**Fig. 4.1** An example of a fire procedure for a health centre.

---

**FIRE PROCEDURES**

(1) If you FIND A FIRE RAISE THE ALARM IMMEDIATELY by breaking the nearest fire glass.
(2) Pick up the NEAREST TELEPHONE and tell the switchboard operator who will call the fire brigade. In the absence of operator, call brigade yourself, stating clearly name, address and telephone number.

On hearing the alarm:

*Doctors*

(1) Leave your consulting room, taking with you any patients.
(2) Go to gathering point for roll call.

*Treatment room staff*

(1) Leave the treatment room, taking with you any patients.
(2) Go to gathering point for roll call.

*Reception staff at the following positions*

**Switchboard:**  **call the fire brigade.**

Reception desk 1:  sweep the corridors clockwise to ensure people have heard the alarm.

Reception desk 2:  sweep the corridors anti-clockwise, as above.

Enquiries:  go to back offices to ensure they have heard the alarm.

Back-up:  go to treatment room to see if any help is needed with immobile patients.

Senior receptionist:  clear the waiting room of people.

*All other personnel*

Leave the building as quickly and orderly as possible.

EVERYONE SHOULD GO TO THE FRONT OF THE CENTRE AND GATHER AT THE RANDOLPH ROAD END OF THE CAR PARK

---

It is unlikely that small surgeries will have trouble with people wandering around their premises. However, larger practices (in particular those housed in health centres) might well not be able to monitor adequately the comings and goings of visitors. An intruder is anyone who is on the practice premises without a legitimate reason for being there. The most likely is the simple trespasser, and since trespass is not a criminal office by itself, the only action that need be taken is to request the person to leave and, if necessary, to escort them off the premises.

If there is any suspicion that the person was intending to commit an offence it is wise to take as many details as possible, such as apparent age and general appearance. When a person is found actually committing an offence, such as breaking in or stealing, then the police should be called immediately. It is worth noting that any citizen has the power of arrest under Sub Sections 2 & 3 of Section 2 of the Criminal Law Act 1967. It is unlikely that managers will wish to take up this option.

Great care should be taken in the use of force. The rule is that only the minimum amount of force necessary to overcome resistance or to repel an attack is lawful. The merest touch may, if the person is offering no resistance or violence, amount to an assault. Particular care must be taken when dealing with children and females, bearing in mind that an allegation of assault is easy to make but difficult to refute. This should be borne in mind when coping with drunks or people acting aggressively.

It is advisable to have lockable rooms or cupboards where staff may keep their personal possessions, such as handbags, whilst they work. It is essential that prescription pads are locked away when doctors leave their rooms. Prescriptions awaiting collection by patients should be kept in a position which is inaccessible to patients, and locked away when the surgery is closed.

## DISPOSAL OF CLINICAL WASTE

From 1 April 1991, the Environmental Protection Act 1990 became law. This puts the onus for the correct disposal of clinical waste onto the producer. In the past general practitioners have been able to blame the carriers of any waste which was not correctly disposed of. The Collection and Disposal of Waste Regulations 1988 (Sl No. 819) defines clinical waste as:

1   any waste which consists wholly or partly of human or animal tissue, blood or other body fluids, excretions, drugs or other pharmaceutical products, swabs or dressings, or syringes, needles or other sharp instruments, being waste which unless rendered safe may prove hazardous to any person coming into contact with it; and

2   any other waste arising from medical, nursing, dental, veterinary, pharmaceutical or similar practice, investigation, treatment care, teaching or research, or the collection of blood for transfusion, being waste which may cause infection to any person coming into contact with it.

Clinical waste must be separate from other waste. The internationally recognized colour for clinical waste bags is yellow. Rigid plastic containers can also be used, and these are preferable for the disposal of sharps. All containers should be clearly labelled as clinical waste, and such waste must be put in secure storage prior to transportation. Black bags should be used for normal office and household waste as this reduces the cost.

In most areas, the FHSA or Health Authority will be making arrangements for appropriate contractors to carry away the waste. Should this not be so, certain very strict regulations apply. Either contact the local council, who will be able to give details of contractors registered with them competent to deal with clinical waste, or the National Association of Waste Disposal Contractors (on 081-824-8882).

A fine of up to £20 000 could be imposed on those who do not meet the required regulations.

## Control of Substances Hazardous to Health Regulations 1988 (COSHH)

Most of these regulations came into force on 1 October 1989. The expression 'substances hazardous to health' covers anything that can harm a person's health, including toxic, harmful, irritant and corrosive substances. Exposing employees to risk and failing to comply with COSHH constitutes an offence and is, thus, subject to penalties under the Health and Safety at Work Act of 1974.

Employees must be informed of any risks arising from their work and of the precautions to be taken. Therefore, it is essential that there is a systematic assessment of:

1   any substances that are present, and in what form;
2   what harmful effects might arise;
3   where and how the substances are handled and used;
4   who could be affected, to what extent and for what length of time;
5   under what conditions;
6   the likelihood that an employee will be exposed; and
7   what actions need to be taken to comply with the regulations.

## CLEANING OF PREMISES

Methods can be used to reduce the time required for day-to-day cleaning of premises. For example, adequate entrance mats reduce the amount of dirt transported into the building. A mat taking six paces reduces the amount of dirt by 50%, and one taking fourteen paces by 80% (Brown 1982). Correct cleaning specifications should be compiled, detailing the frequency and type of cleaning procedures and specifying appropriate cleaning substances and materials. For instance, clinical areas need more frequent and thorough cleaning than do offices; unnecessary applications of polish to certain types of flooring builds up unsightly layers, which need expensive and time-consuming stripping. Care should be taken that non-slip polish is applied; and that when a floor is wet danger signs are evident to prevent accidents.

It is inevitable in surgeries that there will be spillage of body fluids on floors and furnishings from time to time. The availability of suitable cleaning materials for instant use can prevent undue staining. District hospitals have control of infection officers who could be contacted for advice. Regular vacuuming of carpets removes damaging dirt and grit and prolongs their life. Arrangements should be made for periodic deep cleaning.

The monitoring of cleaning standards can take place during the regular inspection of the premises.

## EQUIPMENT

### Medical

A detailed list of treatment room and specialist medical equipment suitable for surgeries is given in the *Practice Nurse Handbook* by K. Bolden and B. Takle (1989).

All equipment should be carefully handled, cleaned, stored and maintained. This can prevent deterioration, serious damage and imperfect performance. Careful attention should be given to the maintenance of ECG machines, defibrillators, cryocauteries and autoclaves. There are special regulations relating to the servicing of autoclaves and to the storage of gas cylinders. The Works Department dealing with local health centres should be able to provide advice to surgeries.

### Other

Adequate office equipment is necessary for staff to accomplish many of their tasks effectively. More and more practices are becoming computerized and there is increased use of information technology, especially for word processing. This is discussed fully in Chapter 6. However, there is still a place for the typewriter, albeit that it might well now be electronic with a memory. It is very difficult to complete detailed forms using a word processor. Some people prefer type-writers and they may be cheaper than word processors.

Shredding machines are useful where it is necessary to dispose of confidential material. Sizes vary from desk top versions to large commercial machines. It should be possible to obtain one that suits the requirements of the practice, or to make arrangements to share the Health Authority's if they have one.

Guillotines are useful for trimming letters when tidying notes in Lloyd George medical record envelopes. Hole punches with measures attached will ensure that the holes appear centrally every time for different size paper, thus ensuring that they are neatly filed in A4 records, or for other similar filing. Useful ideas can be found in brochures produced by local and national office equipment and stationery suppliers.

Furniture and furnishings are important and can enhance the atmosphere of a practice. Pleasant and welcoming reception and waiting areas help create a good practice image. There should be adequate seating arrangements for patients, and, where possible, an area for children to sit or play. A few high seats, preferably with arms, should be available for people who have difficulties in sitting and rising from low seating. There should be space for a wheelchair in the waiting area.

When purchasing desks and chairs for doctors and staff, special attention must be paid to the heights and whether or not castors are advisable. Chairs with adjustable backs and seats are essential for computer operators and typists.

Responsibility for premises and equipment is a very important part of a practice manager's role, one which is often overlooked or downgraded. It should perhaps be given equal importance to finance and people, as it affects or is affected by both. Several Acts of Parliament impose many requirements related to the safety of premises and equipment. The type of decor and state of repair of working surroundings can affect the morale and motivation of staff, and the image of the practice given to patients.

## REFERENCES

Brown E.M. (1982) *Fundamentals of Carpet Maintenance*. Cleaning Research Institute, York.
Bolden K. & Takle B. (1989) *The Practice Nurse Handbook*. Blackwell Scientific Publications, Oxford.

## FURTHER READING

*NHS Estate Management and Property Maintenance*, 1991. Audit Commission, London.

# Chapter 5

# Practice Record Systems

The basic requirement of any office is to have a system for coping with the deluge of information which is constantly arriving. This means that methods have to be devised for handling the information as it arrives and then deciding on an appropriate method of storing it so that it can be easily retrieved. Of course, in general practice the information is often highly confidential and sensitive and this has to be taken into account as well.

By the end of this chapter you will:

1  be aware of the variety of different record systems used in general practice.
2  Be familiar with the issue of confidentiality.
3  Know where to go for further information.

## APPOINTMENT SYSTEMS

Most practices these days run some form of appointment system and patients are increasingly expecting to be seen within a reasonable period of time after their arrival at the surgery. Even those practices with special reasons for running 'open' surgeries, such as rural practices or inner city ones with high ethnic populations, probably benefit from offering at least a proportion of their consulting time by appointment.

An appointment system must be:

1  Realistic.
2  Flexible.
3  Give easy cross referencing.

(1) *Realistic.* There is no point at all in packing patients into a period of time when it is quite impossible for the doctor to see them within that time framework. The doctors (and practice nurses) must decide how frequently they wish to consult and patients should be booked accordingly. A great many training practices now consult at a rate of

about six per hour but eight or ten patients per hour is still not uncommon in non-training practices. It is quite impossible to consult effectively above this rate unless a vast number of consultations are being sought for trivial matters which would be better dealt with in other ways. Also if a doctor is consistently starting his or her surgeries late then he or she will continue to run late all through the session. If this is so it might be better to start booking patients to accommodate his or her timing or discuss with them the problems this is causing for the receptionists.

(2) *Flexibility.* By its nature general practice is never predictable so some flexibility must be built into the system to take account of emergencies and patients defaulting from appointment. This can be a problem but if two patients are booked on the hour rather than one and an emergency box is left every hour or so it will prevent the surgery times becoming too overlong or the doctor waiting for patients to arrive. The alternative is to have an open ended system where all 'extras' are added to the end rather than fitted in. If this system works then patients should be warned that they might have a long wait before being seen.

(3) *Cross referencing.* Many doctors now work closely with practice nurses and often patients will have to be seen by both, for example at a diabetic clinic or for a cervical smear. If confusion is to be avoided then it is best if an overall view of the total appointments for the day can be seen at a glance rather than pages turned or other books consulted. The Lloyd Hammel appointments diary is particularly useful in this respect.

Some enthusiastic computerized practices are experimenting with computer initiated appointments but probably the systems are not yet flexible enough for the average practice.

### Day book

All messages coming to the practice must be recorded carefully, be they requests for visits or other information, and the best way to do this is with a day book.

This is a large book or reference file where all messages are entered under the appropriate doctor. Other members of the primary health care team may also use a message book such as this or, if space allows, the same book. The ideal is that each message is timed and cancelled when read by the recipient. The timing enables a cross check to be made if there is a complaint about a message not being received or acted upon.

It is a good idea to encourage doctors to keep a similar message book at home to record visit requests. This should include the obvious information of name, address, telephone number and problem. The time of receiving and acting on the request should be noted.

## Wall charts and planners

A multitude of these are produced by the pharmaceutical companies or can be purchased. Planners where a whole year is displayed by months is helpful for keeping a check of staff holidays, avoiding overlap and calculating holiday due.

The Department of General Practice in Exeter has produced a wall planner allowing all members of the practice team to keep a check on their training activities and the doctors can total up their PGEA credits. This system is useful because under the 1990 contract staff as well as doctors will be expected to undertake courses.

## PATIENT RECORD SYSTEMS

### Lloyd George medical record envelope

This medical record envelope (MRE) was first produced in 1911, hence its title. It is still the most common form of patient record system and has the advantage of being cheap and taking up relatively little space to store. Its major disadvantages are well known, being the difficulty of writing legible notes on small continuation cards and the bulk produced by folding voluminous letters and reports. However it is quite possible to use this system efficiently, particularly if the notes are regularly pruned, contain a summary card and possibly other cards such as immunization or specific disease record cards (e.g. for diabetes). The requirements of modern practice are increasingly making it more difficult to manage with the Lloyd George envelope, purely because the number of uses of a record are expanding so rapidly and the space is limited.

### A4 folder

In the 1960s and 1970s some enthusiasts introduced the A4 folder which has the immediate advantage of giving far more space for patient details to be entered and the opportunity to display letters and reports in a way that is easily accessible. However, the records are bulky and require a lot of storage space. In addition, unlike the MRE, the practice has to purchase them so that their introduction incurs considerable expense.

## Family folder

Either the MRE or A4 folder may be amalgamated to produce a folder in which the records of a whole family are kept. The advantage is that if a patient enquires about another member of the family, especially a child, the notes are already available. This is particularly valuable when the doctor does not know the patient and their family well. The disadvantage is that the record is again very bulky and requires a good deal of space, both in the filing system and on the doctor's desk.

## Computer

It has been said that any practice wishing to survive into the 1990s will have to computerize at least some part of the record system. This is such an important subject that a whole chapter in this book has been devoted to it and therefore no further discussion will take place here in any detail.

## Specialized registers

### Age/sex register

All practices should now be familiar with the age/sex register as preventive care for children and attainment of cervical smear and immunization targets are almost impossible without one. As the FHSAs are computerized they are offering the facility of an age/sex breakdown to practices and so their information is available. However, if data from the FHSA is queried and arguments ensue then the only basis for this will be reliable practice data.

The earlier age/sex registers have been used from the 1960s onwards. Many of the early ones were in loose leaf book form with each page(s) representing a year. All the patients born in that year were entered on the appropriate page. This system had limitations as pages became scruffy when patients left the practice or died and names were crossed off.

The RCGP then produced age/sex cards, red for females and blue for males. This had a number of advantages. They were easy to store, more information could be entered on the card and the card could be kept even if the MRE had to be returned to the FPC. Computerized age/sex registers have really made the manual systems obsolete but some small practices may still want to use them.

*Disease register*

Apart from identifying the population at risk in a specific age group the age/sex cards could be used to identify certain groups of diseases such as diabetes, asthma, hypertension, etc. This enabled groups of patients to be identified for disease management, such as follow-up, or to be organized into specific clinics, which has been encouraged by the 1990 contract.

Again the manual system has been superseded by the computer which will automatically combine age/sex register, disease register and retrieval systems without the necessity to run them all separately.

## ACCESS AND CONFIDENTIALITY

Medical personnel and professions allied to medicine are constantly reminded during training of the need to respect a patient's right to confidentiality. Office staff will not have had this training and will need to be constantly reminded of it.

Most breaches of confidentiality are not deliberate although gossip, especially in a small town or village, is always a risk of which staff have to be aware. More common faults are:

1 Leaving confidential letters open on the desk while waiting for filing.
2 Having no security system for the records so that any unauthorized person can gain access to them.
3 Answering telephone enquiries without verifying the status of the person making the call.
4 Giving investigation results to a person other than the patient.
5 Answering enquiries from a patient's workplace about their attendance at the surgery.

As can be seen from this list, which is not exhaustive, most breaches of confidentiality arise from thoughtlessness or a desire to be helpful rather than malicious intent. Nevertheless it still leaves the practice open to charges of negligence and the practice manager must be constantly vigilant to see that staff do not fall into careless habits.

Another issue to be resolved is who has access to the patient's record? Obviously any member of staff has an opportunity to see records but formal access by, say, the primary health care team should be discussed and agreed within the practice. The other question to be answered is who writes in the notes? Increasingly all members of the practice may have cause to make entries in the records and, indeed, under the terms of the 1990 contract it would be difficult to avoid doing this. However, entries should be kept to a minimum and the type of entry agreed. Within computerized systems many of these problems can be overcome as the access can be limited by passwords and certain staff can have right of entry to a specific part of the record.

## REPEAT PRESCRIBING

No practice in the UK can easily survive without an efficient repeat prescribing system. The pattern of repeat prescribing is a British phenomenon related to the structure of the NHS. In many countries seeing the doctor will attract a fee and so patients are encouraged to see him or her when the only purpose of the consultation is to collect a regular prescription.

Much has been written about repeat prescribing and the aspects of it related to the doctor/patient relationship. Some doctors will use the system to avoid seeing a patient and some patients use the system as a way of relating to the doctor.

Irrespective of the psychological aspects of repeat prescribing the practice manager is responsible for seeing that the system works well and is not abused. Points to be considered are:

1   The system must be reliable and have a checking mechanism. This means that it should be clear what drugs are involved and when they were last prescribed.
2   It must have a review system. Many repeat prescriptions for everything from cough medicine to major disease treatment can go on for years without being reviewed. This is obviously undesirable as the patient may no longer need the medicine, may be using it inappropriately or have a condition (e.g. hypertension) which is essentially symptomless for most of the time but needs regular review. A stop date is the best way of effecting this. The doctor decides how long it might be appropriate for the prescription to be repeated, e.g. 3 months, 6 months or a year, and this is indicated on the record. When the period has expired the patient cannot get another prescription without a review.
3   It must be secure. In other words the only person with access to the prescription must be the patient or a legitimate representative. Prescriptions should never be left on a notice board in the waiting room or surgery entrance for patients to collect as this inevitably leads to theft.
4   The patient must understand the system and have some form of repeat prescription card upon which details can be entered. The card should also contain details about how to use the system.
5   Telephone requests for repeat prescriptions are common but can lead to a breakdown in the recording system if care is not taken.

Calls are also very time consuming for staff. Wherever possible patients should be encouraged to write or leave their repeat prescription card for collection with a clear indication as to which prescriptions are required. A stamped addressed envelope system can also be encouraged for housebound patients or those unable to get their prescription personally.

6  A computerized system solves all these problems in one action and this was probably the single most useful activity for a computer in the average practice before the 1990 contract. The reduction in staff time spent on filing and paperwork while producing a fail safe method of administration is obvious.

There will be many variations on the office procedures described in this chapter. Indeed new solutions to old problems are constantly being discovered. The practice manager must be aware of all the issues involved and then with the team decide how best to manage them.

## FURTHER READING

Jones R.V.H., Bolden K.J., Pereira Gray D.J. & Hall M.S. (1985) *Running a Practice*. (3rd edition). Croom Helm, London.

Zandler L., Beresford S.A.A. & Thomas P. (1978) *Medical Research in General Practice*. Occasional Paper 5. Journal of the Royal College of General Practitioners, London.

# Chapter 6

# Computers in General Practice

With the arrival of the 1990 contract, a computer system is regarded by many as essential to general practice. It is possible to function adequately without a computer, but procedures that have to be carried out manually are both expensive and tedious. Further, the selection of both hardware and software can be daunting. A computer can considerably enhance the work both clinically and administratively within a practice.

At the end of this chapter you should:

1   Understand the benefits of computerization.
2   Understand some of the pitfalls.
3   Understand some of the issues to consider when obtaining hardware and software.

## BENEFITS OF COMPUTERIZATION

There are five main advantages to a practice of computerization:

1   Access to patient information.
2   Easier repeat prescription systems.
3   Reliable recording of morbidity statistics.
4   Fulfilment of GP terms of service requirements.
5   Improved secretarial work.

### Access to information

Today patients expect rapid responses to requests for information. Most people have become accustomed to easy access of information primarily due to computerized data retrieval systems and they expect no less from the surgery. A system should therefore be able to identify information easily. Most systems couple registration details with an age/sex register enabling staff to identify patients on the list. Patients can be identified by surname and forenames or by other unique identifiers such as a number, date of birth, postcode or NHS number.

## Prescribing

A computerized medical system can automate repeat prescribing. Ideally, it can also generate prescriptions during a consultation. The computer must therefore be fast, easy to use and not too distracting. The advantage of an automated system is that information about drugs prescribed is stored in the patient's computer record thus saving time at subsequent contacts. A protocol must be developed in which the doctor checks the initial drug entries. There need to be subsequent checks to be certain that the patient is not having medication without review, nor is having excess medication, nor medication too infrequently.

The task of issuing the repeat prescription can be delegated to a trained member of staff, who will only need to check with medical practitioners where there has been a change in medication. In dispensing practices, the computer can keep up to date records of stock as well as issuing the script. This helps the practice keep stock at an efficient level, optimizing cash flow.

## Morbidity recording

A good system allows the doctor or staff to enter every contact with the patient. This enables the effective recording of morbidity in the practice. Different systems record morbidity in different ways. The national standard is now the READ system of classification that allows easy entry of data. This system allows searches by category of disease rather than by specific disease name.

## Fulfilment of GP terms of service requirements

Most systems have the ability to record patient encounters, whether in the surgery or elsewhere. This not only helps the practice fulfil its terms of service under the contract, for example screening of those over 75, health checks and so on, but also provides useful monitoring of FHSA claims such as night visit fees. These entries also help provide data for the annual report. Medico-legally, paper entries are still essential if the computer does not have an 'audit trail', an unchangeable record of which doctor saw the patient and the results of the consultation.

### Accounting

Since the introduction of the new contract and budget holding, general practice must be considered a business. Like any other business, it is necessary to keep watch on all aspects of income, expenditure and profit margins. This entails up to date accounting, financial planning and analysis. It seems sensible, if computerized facilities are available, to use the systems for these areas. Computers are an ideal tool for all aspects of financial management. In selecting a system a criterion may be the ability of the computer to run financial packages as well as clinical software. For example, the practice payroll can be computerized, which in a large practice, can save much time for the manager.

## Cash Flow forecasting

Now that the quarterly FHSA statement is fully computerized and details doctors' payments for items of service, fees and allowances, it is possible to predict income. As expenditure is controlled by the practice itself, comparisons can be made between income and expenditure, so allowing the prediction of cash limitation periods. There are several ways of identifying such shortfalls, ranging from sophisticated cash flow accountancy packages to a straightforward spreadsheet. These facilities help the group plan their finances carefully. As part of the concept of financial control, computerized packages will be essential for budget holding practices. All familiar medical software houses have developed systems that enable budget holding practices to monitor and forecast their expenditure accurately.

## Auditing

The new contract requires all practices to produce an annual report. This report must contain various statistics about the performance of the practice, for example consultation rates or out of hours visits. The collection of these data is eased by a computerized system; a manual system could be as efficient but would involve more effort. The content of the annual report is clearly defined, but its layout is not. Software packages such as desktop publishing or graphics make the presentation of the data more appealing, and practices may want to consider whether such software can be operated from their hardware and operating system.

Besides the collection of data for the report there is the need to collect data for auditing. The Medical Audit Advisory Group (MAAG) advises on how to collect this data. A computerized system facilitates retrospective data collection, an almost impossible task without a computer.

**Improved secretarial work**

Office automation is becoming increasingly relevant to general practice. Modern electronic typewriters have sophisticated displays and memories but do not, however, have the ability to perform mail merges. In a mail merge, name and addresses are added to a standard letter (such as a cervical cytology recall letter). This enables the secretary to write to many people easily. If the system also has a relational database, then aspects of a patient's medical history can be copied into a referral letter to a hospital consultant.

## PROBLEMS OF COMPUTERIZATION

Most of the difficulties involved with computerization are not new. Organizations have been tackling the problems shown below since the start of computerization. It is always helpful to seek advice from experienced colleagues or practices using similar equipment. Also, all major software houses have help lines available during working hours. Computer user groups are very helpful and are well worth joining; they consist of individuals interested in particular systems. The groups are organized on a local basis.

There are six main problems for a practice in introducing computerization:

1  Staff attitudes.
2  Financial limitations.
3  Siting limitations.
4  Data protection, security and confidentiality.
5  Training.
6  Choices.

**Staff attitudes**

Many GPs and practice staff have had no experience with computers and a number will see the introduction as a threat. This may partly be due to a fear of the unknown. There may also be a concern that they will not be able to meet the challenge or fully understand new procedures. Computers will change established staff work practices. This needs to be handled sensitively, pointing out the benefits of the system to the staff. One solution is to demonstrate aspects of the system which offer clear advantages such as repeat prescribing. Many staff fear redundancy because of the increasing efficiency, but redundancy rarely occurs as a computer allows for more sophisticated practice and administration.

**Financial limitations**

A practice considering buying equipment will have to find capital to fund the initial purchase. Alternatives are to rent or lease hardware. Additional costs include installation work involving cabling and possible structural alterations. Practices must also budget for training, consumables, licensing and maintenance costs. In normal capital expenditure analysis, cost recuperation would determine the amount available for purchase, but it is difficult to apply this concept to general practice. Financially, it is hard to justify computing in general practice (apart from budget holding practices). In terms of increased efficiency and the reduction of repetitive tasks, a computer can be considered worthwhile.

The best solution is not necessarily the cheapest. History suggests that nearly all systems expand once installed. As a guide, GP computing tends to be more expensive than normal business software because of its specialist nature. It also tends to be packaged with hardware, software, installation, training and maintenance costs in one financial bundle. The government has recognized the problem. The FHSA now funds a percentage of purchasing or leasing, initial staff costs and maintenance costs.

Whether to buy or lease equipment is a difficult decision, as is deciding on which hardware and software to use. The practice accountant can give advice on the financial aspects. Choice of hardware depends on many factors including practice size, whether the equipment is to be used for all patient contacts and so on. Consideration needs to be given to hard disc size (e.g. 80 Mb, 110 Mb), disc access time, type of micro-chip installed (e.g. 386 or 486), computer clock time, ease of connection of peripheral devices and operating system language (e.g. DOS or Xenix). These technical aspects are best discussed with a general practitioner with computer knowledge.

**Siting limitations**

Many systems are not used to their full extent or are branded as difficult. This is usually due to factors not related to the computer itself. A common problem, for example, is bad siting of the equipment. Poor siting can affect system performance or indeed jeopardize security due to possible breaches of confidentiality. Consideration should be given to the following aspects of siting.

*Ergonomics*

The needs of the user should determine the siting of the terminal. The user may have to spend many hours sitting at it. The optimum position for the screen is such that the operator is in a relaxed position with the screen at the best height and distance from their eyes. Strain is caused by glare and reflection from ambient light. Avoid siting screens in direct sunlight. All screens can be adjusted for contrast and brightness. Clean screens regularly with recommended cleansers and encourage operators to adjust the screens to suit their own position. Use comfortable, adjustable chairs with good back support. Noise can affect concentration, so try to site equipment away from the busy front desk yet near enough to consult the screen for information. Avoid using noisy printers in consulting rooms. Many perceive the use of a computer during the consultation as a distraction. Certainly those doctors who are not yet skilled with the keyboard will find entering the data tedious, though a 'mouse' or touch screen will help. Alternatively, data can be entered after the consultation by trained staff.

*Screening from electrical interference*

Some form of interference is common on most network or multi-user systems and is generally caused by external electrical emissions. To counter this, screen data lines within the building. There are, nevertheless, parts of the system which cannot be screened. Magnetic equipment must be kept clear of all data stores, including the hard disc as well as any floppy storage medium. A carelessly placed magnet, however small and innocent, can wipe out months of stored data in a second!

A further problem may arise from infection of the system by a computer virus. This is a piece of program code which copies itself into a part of the hard disc. The effects of viruses are different: many are harmless, but others can destroy data by corrupting or expanding data files. The commonest time for infection to happen is when software is loaded into the machine, but the effect may not be noticed until much later. Reputable software houses do check their software for viruses. Any other software should be regarded as suspect (for example, that borrowed from a colleague). Programs are available that can monitor, or even inoculate, your system for known viruses.

## Data protection, security and confidentiality

Patients expect all personal and private information held on medical records to be kept secure and confidential. This expectation extends to computer data records. The software must guard data from unauthorized access. All systems require password access to both initial entry and different levels of the program. Read and write access should be carefully controlled to ensure that only authorized users enter the data. It is a good idea to change passwords from time to time to preserve secrecy. Data should be protected from unauthorized readers by blanking of screens when not in use. Most software has automatic blanking of screens if no key is pressed for several minutes. Computer terminals should be sited so that information cannot be read by unauthorized people.

Regular copies of changed data should be made. The recommended minimum backup is one set of daily data and one set of weekly data, though practices with larger lists may need to back up more than once a day. The cheapest way of backing up is on to floppy discs, but this is time consuming. A quicker system is on to a tape streamer, or even on to a second hard disc. Copies should be kept in a separate building or in a data-proof safe. Data take a long time to create and can be destroyed in seconds by fire or even by the computer itself. Equipment can be replaced, data cannot. There are firms that may be able to retrieve much of your lost data but at considerable expense.

## Training

With any piece of sophisticated equipment, trained operators work more efficiently than those untrained. It is vital that all computer operators have some degree of training, particularly in the work environment. Managers should look carefully at requirements and decide what level of training is needed and who should attend. 'On-site training' fulfils most needs as it uses the practice's own hardware and software, but tends to be the most expensive. Training courses can also be expensive and unfamiliar equipment is used for practical work. Most package deals include training but this is often limited. Help desks and software support are generally part of maintenance agreements, but supporters may be reluctant to make on-site visits. The most cost effective method is for the practice enthusiast to attend courses. This person then trains the rest of the team, though enthusiasm may need to be tempered with practical application.

## Choices

Choice of computer system remains a difficult area of practice computing. It is wise to learn from other people's mistakes. In general, some guidelines to follow for those practices that have yet to computerize are as follows.

## Software considerations

1 Age/sex register facilities with registration detail that can be easily manipulated to identify patients by using unique identifiers such as name, date of birth, address, NHS number or post code.
2 Clinical records that can be amended and updated to identify patients according to diagnosis, morbidity (preferably using READ codes), target status (cytology and immunization), contraceptive status, and referral status.
3 Patient medication records that include a drug database and allow acute and repeat prescribing with the facility to identify patients by type of drug, compliance and 'repeat until' dates. The system should also provide regular drug updates or allow controlled editing of the drug file.
4 Fast searching, using any search parameter from height and weight through to investigation results. Many systems offer a filter allowing searches on only part of the database.
5 Call and recall facilities for such practice activities as cervical cytology, immunization and health promotion clinics.
6 The ability to handle other software such as a separately purchased word processing or accounts package.

## Hardware considerations

1 Ability to expand the system for future use, for example from single user to multi user, increase in size of hard disks.
2 Enough rear communication ports to connect to modems allowing links to FHSAs, hospitals, pathology laboratories or branch surgeries.
3 Speed of data access.

Some practices may already be computerized but be having difficulties due to such problems as slow access time or slow screen renewal, or even be running out of hard disc space. Further, the software may be inadequate to meet the demands the practice is expecting of it. It is tempting to switch to a new system completely, but this is a very expensive option, as data on one software system are rarely compatible with the format of the new system. It is often possible to build on the existing equipment. Checks must be made to ensure that this is possible under the existing contract with the software suppliers.

## CONCLUSION

There is no doubt that practice computing is here to stay. Computing is no longer the domain of a computer professional. It is now the tool of modern managers. Now is the time for practices to either buy or update computers. The present policy of the Department of Health in providing partial funding will probably be limited in the future. Advantage can be taken of this current concession. Practices who now lease or rent equipment need to consider purchase whilst funds are available. All FHSAs, hospitals and most pathology departments are computerized, and therefore data links or lines will be available for networking to GP surgeries. Computers allow effective and efficient management of a practice. The reality of modern practice is that information technology is essential to the smooth and successful running of a practice.

## FURTHER READING

Fitter *et al.* (1986) *A Prescription for Change.* DHSS, HMSO, London.
Ritchie L.D. (1986) *Computers in Primary Care.* Heinemann, London.
Royal College of General Practitioners (1980) *Computers in Primary Care.* Occasional Paper Number 13. RCGP, London.
Sheldon M. & Stoddart N. (1985) *Trends in General Practice Computing.* Royal College of General Practitioners, London.

# Chapter 7

# Finance

This chapter examines accounting procedures and financial management within a practice. It will enable you to:

1 Effectively record financial transactions.
2 Follow basic accounting procedures.
3 Identify some of the requirements of the PAYE, SSP and SMP systems.
4 Identify how accountants and banks can be of help.
5 Gain further information from appropriate sources.

The sources of income are not explored, and, in particular, no guidance is given on the use of the Statement of Fees and Allowances, 'The Red Book'. This book is written in great detail, is constantly being updated and, where there is any flexibility in interpretation, this can vary in each FHSA or Health Board.

The independent contractor status of general practitioners means that they are self-employed, but contracted to provide medical services. This allows them the freedom to decide how they organize and run their practices. However, they also have the responsibilities associated with running a business as well as the clinical services provided. Their hospital colleagues do not have such freedom, but neither do they have the responsibilities associated with running a business. This is undertaken by their Health Authority.

Practice managers are becoming increasingly involved in the financial management of their practices. Previously many had undertaken such tasks as the recording of payments and receipts, bank reconciliations, and working out salaries and wages under the PAYE scheme. Now they are taking part in the policy making, decision taking and planning. This can involve them in the preparation of a business plan which will have a financial section, and in the preparation of budgets and cashflow analysis. It is often the managers who are liaising with the accountant, bank manager and others concerned with the practice finances. The manager needs to be aware of the best ways of raising money and of investing it. Negotiating skills are necessary for those involved with fund holding and useful when purchasing items of equipment and supplies as well as in non-financial situations.

Whatever the involvement, it is essential that all financial transactions are accurately recorded. It is advisable to have a discussion with the practice accountant about the best way of recording, analysing and presenting the accounts. This should lead to a reasonable bill for the preparation of the end of the year accounts.

For those new to accounting and finance, the following basic procedures are a start to building a system of procedures and controls.

## PAYMENTS

Before making a payment:

1  Check that the goods have been received, or the services provided as invoiced.
2  Check that the invoice is correct. That is, check that the price/s charged is/are as agreed, that the totals are correct, that VAT, if applicable, is correctly calculated.
3  Ensure that the maximum advantage has been taken of the credit time allowed for payment, balanced against any discount for payment within a certain period.
4  Check the method of payment. It may be possible to pay by practice credit card, thus extending the period of free credit.
5  Obtain authority for payment if necessary. Some managers are authorized to make some, or all, payments.

   If making a payment by cheque:

1  Enter all necessary details on the cheque stub: date, payee, amount and invoice number.
2  Enter the cheque number and date paid on the invoice.

## BOOKKEEPING

Many practices have a book-keeper who records the daily financial transactions of the practice. This is sometimes the duty of the practice manager. These transactions should be kept as simple as possible.

1  All money received should be recorded: amount, from whom, for what, date of receipt, date of banking and paying-in book slip number.
2  Money due should be chased up if not received by requested date.
3  Payments out should only be made when duly authorized.
4  Payments out should be recorded: amount, to whom, for what, date and cheque number.

This information can be recorded in several ways, either manually or by using a computer accounting package or spreadsheet.

Cash books are the usual method of recording the receipts and payments made through the bank. Suitable headings for the breakdown of columns should be agreed with the practice accountant. These column headings should be kept under review to ensure that they are not over or under used. Entries in the Sundries column should be kept to a minimum if a comprehensive analysis is to be made of financial transactions.

Entries should be written up from the bank paying-in book (receipts) and from the cheque book (payments). They should be entered in the month that they are paid or received.

To carry out a monthly reconciliation of bank transactions (Figures 7.1 and 7.2):

1  Obtain a bank statement for the month in question.
2  Total all columns in the cash book for both receipts and payments.
3  Tick off in the cash book and on the statement the cheques that

| | Receipts (£) | Payments (£) | |
|---|---|---|---|
| | 2000.00 | | |
| | | 145.60 | |
| | | 550.00 * | |
| | | 1557.00 | |
| | 3150.00 | | |
| | | 50.55 * | |
| | | 16.25 | |
| | 1000.00 † | | |
| | 50.00 † | | |
| Totals | 6000.00 | 2319.40 | as at 30.9.91 |
| Subtract | 2319.40 | | |
| Balance | 3680.60 | | in cash book as at 30.9.91 |

* outstanding cheques not yet presented at bank

| | |
|---|---|
| 550.00 | |
| 50.55 | |
| 600.55 | Total of cheques outstanding |

† receipts not yet banked or showing on bank statement

| | |
|---|---|
| 1000.00 | |
| 50.00 | |
| 1050.00 | Total of receipts not shown on bank statement |

**Fig. 7.1**  Cash book.

|  | (£) |  |
|---|---|---|
| Balance as per bank at 31.8.91 | 3231.15 |  |
| Less outstanding cheques not yet presented | 600.55 |  |
| Plus receipts not shown on statement | 1050.00 |  |
| Equals balance per cash book | 3680.60 * | at 30.9.91 |

* This figure must agree with the balance in the cash book and could be a debit or credit figure.

**Fig. 7.2**   Bank reconciliation.

   have been passed through the bank, and the receipts that have been credited to the account.

**4**   Enter in the cash book any receipts and payments that have not been ticked on the statement. These may be: direct debit and standing order payments, bank account, service and interest charges or bank interest credits, bank transfers, credit transfers from the FHSA or DHA, medical insurance report income, etc.

**5**   Make a list of the cheques outstanding, i.e. those that have not been ticked in the cash book.

**6**   Make a list of any receipts that are not ticked in the cash book.

**7**   Subtract the total payments column from the total receipts column in the cash book, which will give a credit or a debit figure.

**8**   Identify the balance at the bank from the bank statement.

**9**   To this figure *add* the total of receipts outstanding and *subtract* the total of the payments outstanding.

**10**   The resulting figure should correspond with the final balance figure in the cash book. If they do not match a search must be made for the error/s.

Keep a record of these calculations as this monthly bank reconciliation aids the accountant in compiling the end of year accounts and, thus, saves time, which is money, which would have been charged by the accountant.

### Petty cash

It is essential that all receipts and payments are recorded, including those through the petty cash system. Suitable headings should be used in the petty cash book to make these recordings. It is simpler to pay by cheque or credit card as much as possible, as these transactions are then automatically recorded through the cash book. However, it is usual for refreshments, postage and other sundry items to be purchased by cash.

Every time money is drawn from the petty cash a signed note should be made recording the amount, date and signature of the person who has drawn it and received it. When the money is used, receipts should be obtained. The expenditure should be analysed in a similar way to the cash book, e.g. column headings may be Refreshments, Postage, Window Cleaning and others appropriate to practice use.

This cash should be kept in a secure place where there is limited access. Preferably one person should be responsible for the allocation of the money.

## Other cash

Some receipts are in the form of cash, such as payments for: sick certificates, signing of passports, cremation fees, immunization and vaccination certificates for travel abroad, etc. These too should be recorded in a form that can be analysed, with suitable headed columns in a day book. This cash should then be paid into the bank account, being entered in the cash book as a receipt for private fees. All such receipts must be recorded as the Inland Revenue shows a particular interest in such transactions.

## PAYE

The application of the rules relating to payment of employees under the PAYE schemes are fully explained in literature provided by the local Inland Revenue offices. Each partnership will be allocated its own tax reference number, and appropriate documents will be issued according to the number of staff employed. This office will also notify employers of the relevant tax codes for their employees. Anyone new to administering PAYE should contact their local office if they have difficulties. The staff are usually very obliging in giving advice.

## New employees

On joining a practice a new employee, including a trainee general practitioner, should produce:

1  A P45 provided by their previous employers.
2  Their National Insurance Certificate, which will state whether they pay Class A or Class B (married woman) contributions (female employees only).

If they are unable to produce a P45, then a P46 should be completed. This applies to casual employed staff too. Even if staff are paid under the National Insurance Contribution Limited a P46 should be signed and kept by the employer. Students should complete a form P38S.

## Statutory Sick Pay (SSP)

SSP is payable by the employer to all employees over 16 and under 60, for a woman, and under 65 for a man, who are earning a certain level of average weekly pay. The employee must be able to prove that they are ill. It is advisable to ask for this in writing. A self-certificate should be provided for the first week, followed by a doctor's certificate for a longer period of sickness. It is possible for an employer to challenge sickness during the self-certification period if they have reason to believe that the employee is not genuinely sick.

SSP is payable for up to 28 weeks of illness. State benefits take over (if applicable) from this period. The employee should apply to the DSS for these.

Although additional amounts of sick pay are permitted, employers may offset the amount of statutory sick pay against this or against any sick pay they are contracted to pay.

## Statutory Maternity Pay (SMP)

To qualify for SMP a part or full time employee should:

1   Have had 26 weeks' continuous employment.
2   Have normal weekly earnings of not less than the lower limit to qualify for national insurance contributions.
3   Have proof of pregnancy. A MAT B 1 should be sufficient.
4   Have given 21 days' prior notice of intended absence.
5   Be employed on the 11th week before the expected week of confinement.
6   Not work whilst receiving SMP.

SMP is paid for up to 18 weeks and cannot start before the 11th week prior to the expected date of delivery (EDD). The employee must have given up work before the 6th week prior to the EDD. This pay is fully taxable and subject to Class 1 national insurance contributions.

More detailed information on current rules and levels of payment may be obtained from the local social security office who can provide helpful leaflets.

## PROFIT AND LOSS

In compiling the end of the year accounts the accountant will examine the payments and receipts for the year in question. Those that do not relate to that specific year will be extracted. For example, with a financial year ending 30 June: if a telephone bill is paid on 28 June with a standing charge covering the following July to September, this amount will be extracted and carried forward to the next year's accounts; if money is received on 15 July in respect of maternity services provided and claimed before 30 June, this will be extracted and taken into account in the previous year's accounts. Thus, the receipts and payments are converted into the income and expenditure relating solely to the year under review.

By subtracting the expenditure from the income, the true figure of profit or loss for the partnership is arrived at. This profit is divided into the shares appropriate to each partner. The drawings of each partner (including figures paid for superannuation and national insurance from the partnership, which are in effect personal drawings) are calculated for the year. The drawings are then subtracted from the profit allocated, usually leaving an amount over or under paid for that year. This is shown in the end of the year accounts.

## CAPITAL ACCOUNTS

Many people have difficulty in understanding the capital accounts of the partnership. The capital of a general medical partnership covers three areas: property, other fixed assets and working capital. Capital relating to property owned by all, or some of the partners, is the equity that each partner may have at any given year. This will be affected by the share that an individual has in the property, by the property's changing valuation and by the amount repaid on any loan on the property. The other assets include: fixtures and fittings, furniture and equipment (both medical and surgical). The working capital will consist of the money owed to the practice, cash in hand, and the value of stock in hand, such as stationery and dispensing drugs.

## CASHFLOW FORECAST

A useful tool in managing the finances of the practice is a cashflow forecast. Figure 7.3 is an example of such a forecast sheet which was prepared by the AHCPA and the Nat-West Bank Medical Professions Service. The amounts that it is anticipated will be spent and received each month are placed in the Budget columns. Thus, when the monthly budget payments and receipts columns are totalled the net cashflow can be calculated. This will show when cash is likely to be scarce and it may be possible to make adjustments in advance to avoid this. When the exact payments and receipts are known these amounts are placed in the Actual columns and can be compared with the anticipated (Budget column) entries.

**Fig. 7.3**   General medical practice cashflow forecast.

Enter month

Figures rounded to £s

| | Budget | Actual | Budget | Actual | Budget | Actual | Budget | Actual | Budget | Actual | Budget | Actual | Budget | Actual | Budget | Actual | Budget | Actual | Budget | Actual | Budget | Actual | Total Budget | Actual |
|---|---|---|---|---|---|---|---|---|---|---|---|---|---|---|---|---|---|---|---|---|---|---|---|---|
| 1 Capitation fees | | | | | | | | | | | | | | | | | | | | | | | | |
| 2 Other NHS fees/allow | | | | | | | | | | | | | | | | | | | | | | | | |
| 3 Reimb: Anc/Trainees | | | | | | | | | | | | | | | | | | | | | | | | |
| 4 Rent & rates | | | | | | | | | | | | | | | | | | | | | | | | |
| 5 Drugs & appliances | | | | | | | | | | | | | | | | | | | | | | | | |
| 6 DHA reimb | | | | | | | | | | | | | | | | | | | | | | | | |
| 7 Private | | | | | | | | | | | | | | | | | | | | | | | | |
| 8 Other income | | | | | | | | | | | | | | | | | | | | | | | | |
| 9 | | | | | | | | | | | | | | | | | | | | | | | | |
| 10 | | | | | | | | | | | | | | | | | | | | | | | | |
| A Total receipts | | | | | | | | | | | | | | | | | | | | | | | | |
| **Payments** | | | | | | | | | | | | | | | | | | | | | | | | |
| 11 Wages & salaries | | | | | | | | | | | | | | | | | | | | | | | | |
| 12 PAYE/NIC | | | | | | | | | | | | | | | | | | | | | | | | |
| 13 Training | | | | | | | | | | | | | | | | | | | | | | | | |
| 14 Locum/deputizing | | | | | | | | | | | | | | | | | | | | | | | | |
| 15 Drugs/dressings | | | | | | | | | | | | | | | | | | | | | | | | |
| Appliances | | | | | | | | | | | | | | | | | | | | | | | | |
| 16 Rent/rates | | | | | | | | | | | | | | | | | | | | | | | | |
| 17 Repairs/maintenance | | | | | | | | | | | | | | | | | | | | | | | | |
| 18 Services | | | | | | | | | | | | | | | | | | | | | | | | |
| 19 HP/leasing repay | | | | | | | | | | | | | | | | | | | | | | | | |
| 20 Bank/finance charges | | | | | | | | | | | | | | | | | | | | | | | | |
| 21 Loan repayments | | | | | | | | | | | | | | | | | | | | | | | | |
| 22 Accountancy | | | | | | | | | | | | | | | | | | | | | | | | |
| 23 Insurance | | | | | | | | | | | | | | | | | | | | | | | | |
| 24 Motor expenses | | | | | | | | | | | | | | | | | | | | | | | | |
| 25 Drawings | | | | | | | | | | | | | | | | | | | | | | | | |
| 26 Sundries | | | | | | | | | | | | | | | | | | | | | | | | |
| 27 | | | | | | | | | | | | | | | | | | | | | | | | |
| 28 | | | | | | | | | | | | | | | | | | | | | | | | |
| 29 | | | | | | | | | | | | | | | | | | | | | | | | |
| 30 | | | | | | | | | | | | | | | | | | | | | | | | |
| B Total payments | | | | | | | | | | | | | | | | | | | | | | | | |
| C Net cashflow (A-B) | | | | | | | | | | | | | | | | | | | | | | | | |
| 31 Opening bank balance | | | | | | | | | | | | | | | | | | | | | | | | |
| D Closing bank Balance (C-Line 31) | | | | | | | | | | | | | | | | | | | | | | | | |

## WORKING WITH YOUR ACCOUNTANT

It is possible for a manager with financial expertise to compile the end of the year accounts. However, even in these circumstances it is advisable for the practice to engage an accountant, preferably with experience with general medical practice accounts, because they are better able to negotiate with the Inland Revenue regarding the assessment and payment of tax. An accountant will also help with the partners' personal tax matters, and is able to give general financial advice from a personal and a practice point of view.

The accountant should be able to give an impartial opinion on the best ways of borrowing and investing money. This is particularly important when contemplating cost-rent schemes, purchasing computers, cars and other costly items, and in maximizing any income by investing any money surplus to requirements in the long or short term.

When selecting an accountant it is advisable to prepare a list of what services you are expecting to be provided and how much work will be undertaken by the practice. An interview between the prospective candidates, the partners and practice manager is strongly recommended. It is then possible to identify whether or not the accountant is able to provide the appropriate services, how they may be delivered and at what cost. Also, it is equally important that everyone feels confident with, and is able to relate to, the person, or firm, in question. They will be dealing with important matters in respect of the practice and with personal matters relating to the partners.

## WORKING WITH YOUR BANK

A good working relationship with the partnership bank enables a practice manager to obtain a personal service which can help in the running of the practice's bank account and, to some extent, to maximize income and minimize expenditure. Firstly, it is essential to know exactly what the bank charges are for running an account, how much interest is charged for an overdraft, the limit of the overdraft, etc. It is possible to negotiate a reduction in interest or charges if these seem too high, and to waive arrangement fees charged on setting up overdrafts. When negotiating an overdraft it is advisable to ensure that this limit is sufficient to cover all eventualities. Very high charges can be made, without notification, if an account goes above the overdraft limit.

The way practice income is received means that there is likely to be an accumulation of money at certain times in each quarter. A cashflow forecast will identify when these periods are likely to occur. One way of generating income is to ensure that this temporary excess of money is placed in high interest bearing accounts. Some banks have an on-line computer facility which enables the down loading of account information (via a modem) from the bank to the practice computer. A daily check can be made, quickly and easily, of the state of accounts and money transferred appropriately between accounts, via the modem. All this can be accomplished in a matter of minutes, without losing time accessing the appropriate person at the bank, waiting for them to provide the information, requesting the transfer (sometimes a different person), etc.

The banks all have different schemes for lending money, from personal loans to business development loans. When borrowing, it is worthwhile shopping around for the best deal and, if necessary, negotiating with the practice bank manager to see if they are able to match or better it. That is if the practice does not wish to change banks. In changing banks, special arrangements can sometimes be negotiated. However, the work and the aggravation in changing standing orders, direct debits and credits, with some going astray, can outweigh the benefits.

Most banks have special facilities for the payment of practice salaries and wages. These do away with the writing of cheques or individual credit slips, with details usually being entered on one form, and the total amount being debited automatically to the appropriate practice account. This autopay facility can also, in some cases, be accessed via a computer modem.

## FURTHER READING

Dean J. (1990) *Making Sense of Practice Finance*. Radcliffe Medical Press, Oxford.
*The Business Guide for Medical Practices*, produced annually by Touche Ross & Co., 112 High Street, Croydon, CRO 1ND, telephone 081-680-4647.
Conservation of Energy costs. Financial Pulse, 4 December 1990.
Social Security Pensions Act 1975.
Transfer of Undertakings (Protection of Employment) Regulations 1981, from the Department of Employment.
Social Security and Housing Benefits Act 1982.
For PAYE – contact 'Inland Revenue' in local telephone directory.
For National Insurance – contact 'Social Security, Department of' in local telephone directory.

# Chapter 8

# Employment

This chapter highlights the particular areas that should be given careful consideration in the employment of staff and should enable you to:

1  Analyse your requirements for a new member of staff.
2  Plan how to recruit and select a suitable member of staff.
3  Understand the laws relating to employment and to health and safety.
4  Learn where to obtain further information on the employment of staff.

Managing people is an important part of a practice manager's role, and is sometimes the part that causes the most difficulties. The recruitment and selection of the right people for the right job should be a sound basis on which team building can flourish. However, this is not easy to achieve. A beginning is to ask the following questions when a vacancy occurs, or new tasks need doing. Is a new employee really needed? Could work be redistributed, or someone else take over the job, whose own workload has reduced? Good manpower planning ensures effective use of human resources. It may give the opportunity for a review of all staff, their hours and the work undertaken.

On reaching the decision to employ a new member of staff, it is advisable to compile the following three documents: a job analysis; a job description; a person specification.

## JOB ANALYSIS

Some questions that need to be answered are:

1  What needs to be done and why does it need to be done?
2  Where is it to be carried out?
3  How is it to be carried out?
4  To whom is the person to be responsible?
5  For whom is the person to be responsible?

6   For what is the person to be responsible?
7   With whom will they have to relate, internally and externally?
8   What standard of performance is required?
9   What qualifications, training, experience and skills are required?
10  What is the required state of health?
11  Check with the person who currently holds the job, unless it is a new post.

This is a suggested list and there may be other questions that are appropriate to be answered. It will be useful to check with the person who is currently undertaking the job and obtain their view. Discussions with other members of the team may also affect decisions on the job to be done.

## JOB DESCRIPTION

On completing the job analysis it will be possible to draw up a job description. Although there is no standard model for this, the following example can be adapted for individual use.

*Title of job:* senior medical receptionist.

*Responsible to:* the practice manager.

*Responsible for:* four part time receptionists; a filing clerk; a telephonist. The appointments book; the filing system and medical records. The switchboard.

*Main purpose of job:* to ensure the smoth running of the reception area in order to provide an optimum standard of service to patients.

*Main duties:*

Patients:

1   To ensure a friendly welcome to all patients and visitors.
2   To answer patients' queries, book appointments, take messages efficiently, and offer the most effective service possible.
3   To respond to any complaints patients may make by referring them to the practice manager, or a doctor, if it is not appropriate to deal with it personally.

Doctors:

1   To provide an effective service to doctors to enable them to give a high standard of care to patients.

Staff:

1 To arrange and manage the staff rota to ensure adequate cover of the reception.
2 To organize the holiday rota and to arrange cover for holidays and sickness.
3 To supervise the staff when carrying out their duties, to ensure that they maintain the required standard of performance.
4 To deal with any problems that may arise, and to refer them to the practice manager when appropriate.

Systems:

1 To ensure that the appointments book is maintained to the required standard, and to liaise with doctors on the date and times of their surgeries.
2 To ensure that all visits are logged accurately in the visits book, and to supervise the logging of all messages received in reception.
3 To maintain the filing systems for medical records, letters, reports, etc.
4 To supervise the checking, recording and dispatching of all FHSA claim forms.
5 To open and distribute all incoming mail and to arrange the recording and dispatching of outgoing mail, both internal and external.

Reception:

1 To maintain this area in a clean and tidy manner.

The above is just an example of some of what might be included in a job description for a senior medical receptionist. It is not meant to be an authoritative description.


## PERSON SPECIFICATION

It is then necessary to have a clear idea of what kind of person is required to fit the job description. The areas that might be addressed are:

*Physical factors*

1 Tidy appearance.
2 Intelligible speech.
3 Good hearing.
4 Over the age of 21 and under the age of 50.

5   Good health, with no history of illness that might be related to, or lead to, drug abuse.
6   Friendly and cheerful manner.

*Education, qualifications, experience and training*

1   'O' levels in English and mathematics.
2   Previous experience of working as a receptionist, preferably in general practice.
3   To have had at least a year's experience of supervising people.
4   To be prepared to undertake training, sometimes out of working hours.

*General intelligence, personality and adaptability*

1   To be motivated to work with a team in a busy, sometimes stressful, environment.
2   To show evidence of ability to lead team when necessary.
3   To be able to work flexible hours.

*Special aptitudes*

1   To be articulate and numerate.

*Personality*

1   To have pleasant disposition, be confident, and reliable.

*Other circumstances*

1   To live within reasonable distance of the surgery.
2   To have no criminal convictions.

It should also be recorded as to which items of the specification are desirable and which are essential. The above requirements will vary according to the details of the job description. They should be as precise as possible to aid the process of selection.


## ADVERTISING

The wording of the advertisement is crucial. Precise, but detailed, requirements will cut down the number of inappropriate applicants, and attract those who might be most suitable. The details will be taken from the job description and person specification which have been prepared, and might include:

1   The name and address of the practice.
2   The title of the job.
3   A brief statement of what the job entails.

4 Qualifications and experience required.
5 The age range.
6 The salary range and any special benefits.
7 How to apply and the closing date for applications.

The advertisement could be placed in the local Job Centre and local paper. Some FHSAs will place advertisements in their bulletins. Employment agencies can be used, but these are sometimes very expensive. It is advisable to ask for a handwritten application together with a *curriculum vitae*, although a comprehensive application form may make the latter unnecessary. It will be immediately evident from the application whether or not the writing is easily legible.

## SELECTION

Initial weeding out of unsuitable candidates can be done from the applications. An invitation to an informal interview can be made to those on the first short list. At this interview the applicant can be introduced to as many of the team as possible, and spend time with the people with whom they may be working. A tour of the premises and a discussion of what is involved in the job on offer can give them an excellent idea of the demands that may be made upon them and the surroundings in which they will be working. A second short list can be made of candidates to attend a formal second interview.

For the formal interview it is necessary to plan effectively in order to get the best out of the interviewee:

1 Who will be present, and who will lead the interview.
2 What questions will each person ask. This is best divided into areas such as: personal; education, qualifications and experience; motivation; leisure activities and interests; reasons for leaving or wanting to leave, current job (if applicable) and for making the application for job on offer.
3 What, if any, tests will be carried out.
4 Where will it take place, and how will the furniture be placed.
5 Who needs what paperwork at the interview.

It is important to ensure that open, as well as closed questions are put to the candidates. The closed question will ensure a precise answer to a specific question, such as 'how long did you work in your previous job?' An open question should encourage the person to talk more freely and express their views, i.e. 'What did you feel about the work you did there?'

If planned effectively there will be no difficult silences with everyone waiting for someone else to ask a question. The interview should flow smoothly with the candidate talking for most of the time. The actual selection should be made by the interviewers matching the interviewees to the person specification.

It is preferable to have a team which is well balanced in its composition and this will need to be taken into consideration when selecting a new member of the team.

When employing staff it is essential that notice is taken of relevant details of the following Acts of Parliament:

Equal Pay Act 1970
Health and Safety at Work etc. Act 1974
Congenital Disabilities (Civil Liability) Act 1976
Sex Discrimination Act 1975
Race Relations Act 1976
Employment Protection (Consolidation) Act 1978
Employment Act 1980
Employment Act 1982
Social Security Act 1986
Equal Opportunities Act 1988
Employment Act 1989

## CONTRACT OF EMPLOYMENT

A detailed job description provides a sound basis on which to build an employee's working practices and also interpersonal relationships. A legal contract exists from the time a job is offered and accepted and is not restricted to the written word. Oral agreements after commencement of work and common practices form part of the contract.

A written contract of employment must be provided within 13 weeks of an employee starting work except in the following circumstances:

1   Anyone who is not an employee, for example, an agency medical secretary.
2   Employees who are normally employed less than 16 hours a week, unless they have been employed continuously by their employer for at least 8 hours a week for at least 5 years.
3   An employee who is re-engaged on the same terms whose period of employment ended with the same employer within the previous 6 months.

Model contracts can be provided by local British Medical Association offices and AHCPA. Other relevant booklets are those produced by the Department of Employment and the following details are extracted from these.

The written contract should include:

1 Name of employer.
2 Name of employee.
3 Date of commencement of employment and whether any employment with a previous employer counts as part of the employee's continuous period of employment, and if so the date on which that period of continuous employment began.
4 Title of job.
5 The scale or rate of pay, including overtime rates, and intervals between payments, that is, monthly, weekly or some other period.
6 Terms and conditions relating to:
  (a) Hours of work.
  (b) Holidays, including Bank Holidays.
  (c) Holiday pay and entitlement.
  (d) Incapacity for work due to sickness or injury, including sick pay.
  (e) Pensions and pension schemes, except where employees are covered by statutory pension schemes and their employers already provide this information.
  (f) The length of notice for termination of employment which the employee must give and is entitled to receive. If the contract is for a fixed term, the date when this contract expires.

If there are no terms for any of the above items then the contract should state this, e.g. no pension settlement.

The written statement must contain details of disciplinary rules, disciplinary and grievance procedures and appeals. For employees to meet the criteria for receiving such a statement they must have:

● started work before 26 February 1990; or
● started work on or after 26 February 1990 where the employer has 20 or more employees; or
● where a firm expands beyond 19 employees, the twentieth and every subsequent employee acquires this right.

Thus, those who are not entitled to such details are:

1 Employees who started work after 20 February 1990 where the employer has 19 employees or fewer.
2 Anyone who is not entitled to a written statement.

However, it is good practice to include such details on a voluntary basis, and an employee must still be given the name of the person to whom they should go with a grievance.

The additional note must:

1    Specify any disciplinary rules, except those relating to health and safety at work (which should be in a separate document).
2    Detail the person to whom the employee should go, and how this should be effected, if dissatisfied with a disciplinary decision, or for seeking a redress of any grievance relating to his or her employment.
3    Explain if any further steps follow from such an application.
4    State whether a contracting-out certificate under Social Security Pensions Act 1975 is in force for employment in respect of which the written statement is being issued.

Any of the above can be provided in a separate document, providing the employee has easy access to it.

If there are any changes in the terms of employment the employer has to inform the employee within 1 month of its introduction in writing, unless up to date reference documents are kept. Then it is the reference document that must be updated within 1 month.

Circulars may be used or reference documents pinned to notice boards. However, these must be kept for reference purposes and information as to where they can be accessed included in the written statement.

### Complaints concerning written statements

If an employee has not received a written statement he or she may apply to an industrial tribunal. The tribunal may then decide what details the written statement should have included.

A tribunal cannot make judgement on disputes about failure to observe the terms of service. Either the employer or employee may bring an action in the civil courts of law if satisfaction cannot be gained in any other way.

## EMPLOYMENT RIGHTS FOR THE EXPECTANT MOTHER

These rights are set out in the Employment Protection Consolidation Act 1978, and have been amended by the Employment Acts in 1980 and 1982 and the Social Security Act 1986.

The three main rights an expectant mother acquires are:

1    Not to be unreasonably refused time off for antenatal care and to be paid when permitted that time off.
2    To complain of unfair dismissal because of pregnancy.
3    To return to work with her employer after a period of absence on account of pregnancy or confinement.

Women who are not employees are not covered by these Acts.

Full details can be found in the Department of Employment's booklet 'Employment rights for the expectant mother'.

## WRONGFUL DISMISSAL

Most employees are entitled to receive laid down periods of notice:

1  One week's notice after 1 month's service.
2  Two weeks after 2 years' service.
3  An additional week for each complete year of employment up to 12 weeks for 12 years' of service.

If appropriate notice is not given, or pay in lieu of notice, it could be construed that the employee has been wrongfully dismissed.

## UNFAIR DISMISSAL

The definition of unfair dismissal is the termination of employment by:

1  The employer, with or without notice; or
2  the employee's resignation, with or without notice, where the employee has resigned because the employer is in breach of contract or has behaved in a manner leading to constructive dismissal; or
3  the expiry of a fixed-term contract without its renewal; or
4  the employer has refused to allow an employee to return to work after the birth of her baby for which she is legally permitted to do so.

The following people cannot complain of unfair dismissal:

1  Those who are not employees.
2  Employees who have not completed 2 years of continuous employment, except for those employees taken on before 1 June 1985 (where there are more than 20 employees). They need only have completed 1 year of continuous employment.
3  Employees who work less than 16 hours a week unless they have been employed for at least 8 hours a week for at least 5 years.

## FAIR DISMISSAL

An employer can justify fair dismissal for the following reasons:

1  Related to the employee's capability or qualification for the work.
2  Related to the employee's conduct.
3  Redundancy.

**4**   Statutory duty or restriction.
**5**   Some other substantial reason which could justify dismissal.

Further details can be found in the Department of Employment's booklet 'Unfairly dismissed?'

## REDUNDANCY

After 2 years' continuous service employees are entitled to redundancy payments, which depend upon the number of years of service and the individual's pay.

For a person to be made redundant their job should have disappeared. This may arise because an employer has been forced to reduce the work-force, a work-place is closing down, or fewer workers of a particular kind are needed, or expected to be needed. If an employer immediately engages a direct replacement, this is not redundancy. However, there is not a problem if the employer is recruiting staff of a different type, or for a different location, unless the contract of a dismissed employee requires them to move to a new location.

If there is a need to reduce the work-force, an employee(s) may move into a different job(s), or jobs from which a person (people), has been dismissed. As long as vacancies are left elsewhere in the business, and there is a net loss of jobs, the dismissed employee(s) may still qualify for redundancy payment(s).

Certain employees who have been dismissed through redundancy are entitled to time off with pay, during working hours, to look for another job or to make arrangements for training in order to find suitable employment. The employee should be paid at the normal hourly rate for such absence, but not more than two-fifths or a week's pay, irrespective of the time off allowed.

Some of those employees who may not qualify for redundancy payments are:

**1**   An employee whose service ends on, or after, their 65th birthday.
**2**   An employee whose contract, or practice policy, states an earlier retiring age, and who has reached that age.
**3**   An employee on a fixed-term contract of 2 years' or more duration, who has agreed in writing that redundancy payment should be waived if their service ends before the agreed term.
**4**   An NHS employee who is covered by some other agreement.

If there is a dispute about redundancy payment this can be referred to an industrial tribunal. Although this can be done at any time, the right to payment may be lost if the employee has not taken appropriate steps. In certain cases, under special circumstances, the tribunal may still consider payment after 6 months.

## ANTI-DISCRIMINATION LEGISLATION

It is unlawful for employers to discriminate:

1 On grounds of sex or against married persons.
2 On grounds of race, colour, nationality or ethnic or national origins.
3 Against equal pay, terms and conditions of service. This applies to like work of similar value undertaken by men or women.
4 Against an employee who belongs to a trade union or against an employee who does not belong to a trade union.

Discrimination means the less favourable treatment of someone on specified grounds. This also includes the application of requirements or conditions which may have a disproportionate detrimental affect on a person, or a group of people, and the victimization of someone who has made a complaint under these Acts.

Exceptions are for practices with fewer than six employees, but this exclusion does not apply to victimization.

## REHABILITATION OF OFFENDERS

The 1974 Rehabilitation of Offenders Act allows a specific 'rehabilitation' period after a person is convicted. If no further offence is committed during this period the conviction becomes 'spent' and the person is 'rehabilitated'. They do not have to declare this on the application form for a job. However, this Act does not apply to the NHS and this fact should be mentioned on job application forms. That is, it is lawful to ask whether or not an applicant has ever had a criminal conviction.

## HEALTH AND SAFETY AT WORK etc. ACT

The main part of health and safety legislation is covered in Chapter 4. Employers are responsible for the welfare of their directly employed staff, as well as their health and safety. However, for most health centre managers, whilst they are responsible for the 'health and safety' aspects of the premises and equipment, they are not concerned with the welfare of the primary health care team working in the centre but who are managed by other NHS personnel.

The welfare aspect of employment is sometimes hard to define, but certainly includes appropriate cloakroom and refreshment facilities for staff. It is important for the well-being of employees that the environment is as pleasant as possible, that a reasonable temperature is maintained, and there is sufficient ventilation and lighting so that staff may be comfortable and able to give an optimum work performance.

## CONGENITAL DISABILITIES ACT

This Act requires female employees to notify the employer of pregnancy once it has been medically confirmed. This enables employers to take appropriate action to ensure that the member of staff is not exposed to any dangers that could adversely affect the unborn child. This could apply to a practice nurse who may be seeing patients with infectious diseases, or to a cleaner who may be using inappropriate equipment. This act does not in any way infringe the entitlements to leave and pay incurred by a pregnancy.

## INSURANCE

In these days of increased violence in society it is advisable to take out insurance to provide cover in the event of employees being assaulted whilst at work. Such premiums are not expensive.

By law a certificate of employer's liability should be displayed publicly where it can be seen by all staff. Such liability often comes as part of a package including the surgery buildings and/or contents' insurance policy.

It is important that managers keep abreast of laws relating to employment. Many potential problems can be avoided if appropriate actions have been taken to ensure that all parties know their rights and responsibilities.

## FURTHER READING

Ellis N. (1990) Employing staff. *British Medical Journal.*

Booklets are produced by:

ACAS
BMA, Tavistock Square, London, WC1H 9JR.

Other useful free booklets produced by the Department of Employment are:

*Rights to notice and reasons for dismissal*
*Procedure for handling redundancies*
*Suspension on medical grounds under health and safety regulations*
*Itemized pay statement*
*Time off for public duties.*

Chapter 9

# Communication Systems

Electronic and telephonic communication systems have made tre-
mendous strides in the last few years. They can considerably ease the
passing of information from one place to another and practices should
give thought as to how they might wish to avail themselves of these
facilities. It is not the intention in this chapter to cover all the options
in detail but to give the reader some idea of what is available. By the
end of the chapter you should:

1  Be aware of modern telephonic developments.
2  Have enough information to decide whether any of these developments would be of interest to your practice.
3  Know where to go for further information.

## SURGERY TELEPHONE SYSTEMS

It is likely that the size of the partnership, number of patients, and type
and number of staff will determine the type of telephone system that
is needed. For smaller practices it is not necessary to have a
switchboard and telephone operator. British Telecom and Mercury
Communications offer systems which allow the linkage of a small
number of terminals, but which have highly advanced facilities. These
include auto-dial keys, call divert, pick-up groups, hands-free operation, messaging, paging and conference calls.

Larger surgeries and health centres will need many lines and
terminals, with a switchboard and operator competent to work the
sophisticated computerized systems that are available. For a very busy
practice, call sequencing is advisable so that patients' calls are queued
and answered in turn. Some models offer a message and/or music
whilst patients are waiting to be put through.

## MOBILE TELEPHONE SYSTEMS

Main systems use the Cellnet or Vodaphone networks. Both systems
cover over 97% of the British population, and have enhanced service

on the principal motorways. There are three forms of mobile telephone: the transportable, the hands free in-car, and the transmobile.

Hand portables are suitable for use in built-up areas and on main motorways and trunk roads. However, their power is limited, so only moderate coverage can be offered. It is possible to buy kits which allow the phone to be installed into a vehicle to take advantage of 'hands free' calling, and a power booster which allows the phone to be more powerful in rural areas.

Transportable phones are larger, than hand portables, but they are more powerful by comparison. The advantage in opting for a transportable cellphone is the ability to take advantage of the maximum cellular coverage offered in the United Kingdom, but with the flexibility of not being tied to your vehicle. It is unlikely that this kind of coverage will be needed just for surgery use.

In-car mobile phones are designed to be used while driving. They have a 'hands free' facility that allows the user to make a call legally whilst driving. Most mobile cellphones have an option to convert into a transportable unit, which is probably the most useful combination for a general practitioner.

Sets will either re-charge in the car or on a trickle charge at home or in the surgery. Some cellphones are small enough to fit neatly in the pocket.

Both British Telecom and Vodaphone offer a messenger service. Calls can be diverted to a message taking facility, either when the phone is unattended, or if a call is not answered within a specified time. This is particularly useful if the phone is used where reception is variable. In a poor area, the call is automatically diverted to the answer machine.

## ANSWER MACHINES

Answering machines are commonly used in a surgery after it has closed. They are connected to a telephone terminal and the patient's call is picked up by the machine, a message plays giving information of where the patient should telephone to speak to a doctor or a person able to help them. This is not the best method of dealing with out-of-hours calls, as it involves the patient in the cost and trouble of making two calls and of recording the second number to be dialled. This may not be easy for a distressed person.

Many models can be remotely accessed to either pick up messages or change the outgoing message. Some record the number of calls that have been received, and new models will indicate the date and time of the call.

## CALL FORWARDING

One of the options offered by this British Telecom service is Customer Controlled Forwarding. This service is connected to the surgery telephone number and can be switched on and off at will from any other phone. On leaving the surgery a code is dialled to set up the Call Forward and all calls will be redirected to the number of your choice. This service can be set up at a distance. This service is much more acceptable to patients than having their call answered by an answering machine, where they then have to dial another number. One disadvantage is that the practice pays the cost of the diverted call.

A similar service is provided in new electronic exchanges by 'Star Service'. Calls can be diverted to any number in the world, the subscriber to the telephone paying the extra charge. Other facilities included in this system are call waiting indication, call costing and barring of outgoing calls.

There are a multitude of telephone systems offering a complexity of services. Computerized switchboards allow visual monitoring of which terminals and lines are in use, the number of calls stacking, the metering of units used at each terminal, the barring of non-local and/ or international calls, the production of reports on use, conference calls, and interrupt facilities which can be used in emergencies, to name just a few options. Terminals have number storing and call diversion facilities.

Terminals can be set in groups so that if a phone rings in one part of the reception, by dialling a code at another terminal it will pick up that call. This is a very useful facility in a large reception area, when perhaps someone has temporarily left their post. Their colleague does not have to move away from their work station to pick up the call.

## PAYPHONES

Many surgeries have found the installation of payphones a useful service for the patients. It can cut down on demands on the receptionists for telephoning for taxis or friends to pick up patients. If a surgery is situated in an area without a payphone, it could be that members of the public come to the surgery specifically to make use of this service. This has its advantages and disadvantages, much depending on where the payphone is situated within the building. It can be very intrusive to have people chatting loudly on a phone close to the reception desk, but it can also be a source of income. Payphones are not always profitable and appropriate research should be carried out into potential usage if it is necessary for the phone to be profit making.

Some taxi companies will install telephones with a free direct line to their company. This is useful if your patients are large users of taxi services.

## FACSIMILE MACHINES

More surgeries are installing fax machines. The advantages are the speed of transmission of text, graphs, photographs and other documents. It can take as little as 17 seconds to send an A4 sheet, and the fax is charged at the cost of telephone calls so that faxes can be sent cheaply at off-peak times. There does not have to be somebody at the other end of the line to take the call. In the past a disadvantage was that fax paper was waxed, flimsy and the ink tended to fade with time. Now there are plain paper faxes. Most have a guillotine which cuts the pages being received to the length of the pages being transmitted. Many hospitals, FHSAs and surgeries are communicating via this medium.

## PAGING FACILITIES

Radiopagers are perhaps the commonest method of doctors keeping in touch with their surgeries. By dialling a designated number a bleep in the pager is activated notifying the doctor to call the surgery. Some bleeps have different tones indicating whether or not the call is urgent, others have visual displays which give messages. The bleep can be switched onto 'hold', whereby it does not bleep but stores the call until reactivated.

Both British Telecom and Mercury Communications offer a range from sleek, pen-shaped pagers, to larger versions offering a 90 characters message display.

BT's Message Link service allows you to link your pager to BT's Voice Messaging service. People simply call your personal Message Link telephone number from anywhere, listen to your recorded greeting and leave their spoken message at any time. Message Link will then page you and, by using your own identification number, you can then listen to your messages. This is not a facility that will be used for emergency medical situations, but it may have a use for other communications between surgery and distant doctor, or doctor and home.

## TELEPHONE ANSWERING SERVICES

The best known organization offering a telephone answering service is Health Call (previously Air Call). Calls are diverted from the surgery, either directly or via an answer phone, to Health Call offices where nurses trained to take and assess calls deal with the patients' requests. The practice duty doctor is then bleeped. This doctor contacts Health Call for the message, a useful facility where a doctor does not have someone at home to answer the telephone.

## ELECTRONIC COMMUNICATIONS

By using a modem with a computer it is possible for computers to 'speak to one another'. This allows a high speed exchange of data. For a few years some banks have been offering this facility. For example, National Westminster Bank have at times offered their Bankline service at a special rate for medical practices. The latest information regarding your bank accounts can be downloaded daily, so there is no waiting for bank statements which can be printed immediately. Money can be transferred from a current account to a high-interest account at the touch of a few keys. It can be transferred back, equally quickly and easily, thus allowing the maximum interest to be made. Messages can be sent to the bank, for example ordering cheque or paying-in books.

BT's Telecom Gold service allows you to key in your message and where you want to send it in the Telecom Gold network – your words go directly to the 'mail box' of the person you specify. This allows a two-way flow of messages. There is also a large library of business information that you are able to access. This may be an alternative way chosen by some practices of communicating between practices, the FHSA, Health Authorities and others.

British Telecom, via Prestel, have both an electronic Yellow Pages and directory enquiry services. It is possible to access up-to-date comprehensive national classified information via a PC with a modem using Prestel.

## VIDEO CONFERENCING

Both British Telecom and Mercury offer this service. It enables meetings to be held at a distance and cuts down travelling costs. This service allows the transmission of 35 mm slides, high resolution graphics and other inputs, as well as the ability to see one another whilst talking. BT have centres with conference rooms equipped with cameras and monitor screens. With Mercury no dedicated studio facilities are necessary. In the future it is possible that this facility will be used for training purposes as well as for meetings. It could cut down not only on the cost of travel, but of time and wear and tear associated with 'getting away' from the surgery.

## VOICE MESSAGING SERVICE

Mercury's service allows you to send and receive spoken messages at any time, via any direct dialling public telephone service. Your message is stored on computer disk for delivery to the right person or persons. You receive messages when you choose, rather than suffer interruption from telephone calls. It will re-direct, save or delete messages.

## THE DUOPOLY

When the government created a duopoly by allowing a second service, Mercury Communications, to compete with British Telecom for some services and goods, it became possible to reduce the cost of some calls. Mercury offers significant cost savings of up to 20% on non-local calls or fax transmissions. For some practices, this may be important as they may work with hospitals, FHSAs, Health Authorities and other bodies outside their immediate locality. Furthermore, Mercury charges only for the exact duration of your call instead of rounding-up the charge to the next time unit. Their bills are fully itemized showing date, time, duration, charge, destination number, and town of call. It is possible to allocate outgoing calls to three charge numbers when dialling, which are shown as three separate totals on the account. All these are useful checks on the use of the telephone in the surgery.

The Mercury 'Smart Box', or 'Access 2200 Box' device automatically divert calls via the cheapest route, whether that is BT or Mercury. In several locations in the UK Mercury works with local Cable TV Operations to provide an advanced telecommunications service. The Mercury/Cable Operator alliance allows medium to small businesses to gain direct digital connection to the Mercury network. This gives significant cost savings on all calls, including local ones.

## PHOTOCOPIERS

A photocopier is no longer a luxury in a practice, but a necessity with the increasing demand for retaining copies of, say, medical reports, some of the new forms associated with the new contract, annual reports and business plans.

The range is vast, from desk-top to collating, double-sided large models. The volume of copies determines the minimum standard of machine needed, followed by selecting other facilities of particular use to the practice. This may be a reducing and enlarging facility, the ability to use different colour toners, or the automatic selection of paper from several different paper size cassettes loaded in the machine. Some machines allow the copying of pages of large books laid flat on the platen.

Care should be taken in negotiating the acquisition of copiers, as the cost per copy can vary enormously whether or not you are leasing, renting or buying the machine.

For more detailed information on services and products contact:

British Telecom – dial 100 and ask for 'Sales Information'.
Mercury Communications – dial 0800 424 194.

## FURTHER READING

Herd A. (1991) Photocopiers. *Medeconomics* **12** (9). Haymarket Publications, London.
*The BT Business Catalogue* (1991) British Telecom plc, London.
*A Guide to Services* (1991) Mercury Communications Limited London.

# Chapter 10

# Training Practices

## HISTORY

The training of general practitioners for their role has altered out of all recognition in the past 20 years. Up to 1951 it was not even compulsory to do a pre-registration year as a houseman and many doctors entered general practice without adequate or appropriate training.

By the end of the chapter you should:

1 Understand the training requirements for a career in general practice as a principal.
2 Be familiar with the preparation required to become a training practice.
3 Understand the issues involved in having a trainee GP in the practice.

After the NHS was established in 1948 a 1-year apprenticeship type training was introduced on a voluntary basis. For about a decade this was fairly widely used as a way of giving employment to doctors returning from the forces while they looked for a practice. There was no formal training component to this trainee year and practices who entered the scheme were not adequately assessed or trained for the educational responsibilities.

As the struggle to find a practice became easier in the early 1960s this apprentice training with its overtones of cheap labour fell into disrepute and the system withered away as fewer doctors were interested in the arrangement.

A rejuvenation of training for general practice occurred in the early 1970s as the first formal vocational training programmes began to be estabished in response to the Todd Report of 1968 on postgraduate medical training. Throughout the 1970s the number of vocational training programmes for general practice increased rapidly and formal training as a discipline was eventually established by the Vocational Training Act of 1982. Since that time no new entrant to practice has been able to become a principal without undertaking a minimum 3-year training programme, of which 1 year has to be in an approved training practice. The approval of a practice for training purposes is now a formidable procedure and requires considerable preparation on the part of practice and partners before it is given.

## WHY HAVE A GP TRAINEE?

### Benefits

1   Many doctors have some interest in teaching and passing on their skills to others. They may have students in the practice, run evening first aid classes, and so on. The ultimate challenge is to have a young doctor on the threshold of his/her career working with you for up to a year as a preparation for their lifetime's work. The one to one relationship during this time is such that lifelong friendships are often forged.
2   There is no doubt that training practices do have to achieve a high standard and as such are recognized by their peers. Some practices will wish to train both to have their standards measured and to be recognized formally as offering high quality care.
3   Treading the fine line between giving a trainee enough work for him/her to obtain adequate clinical experience without being exploited as an extra pair of hands is extremely difficult. In general terms the practice should still be able to function adequately without the workload being such that the trainee's contribution is absolutely necessary. Some of the clinical workload carried by the trainee should compensate for the time spent by the trainer on teaching activities. Nevertheless, having a trainee in the practice does make it easier to cope with unexpected extra demands such as a flu epidemic or the sudden illness of a partner.
4   Young doctors who have recently undergone training and left the hospital environment will often bring new ideas and perspectives to the practice.
5   It is a common phenomenon in general practice that after some years doctors begin to look for other stimulating outlets. The challenge of training is often the catalyst required to recharge the batteries of enthusiasm amongst the partners and this function should never be underestimated.

### Disadvantages

1   There is no doubt that the preparation of a practice for training and the process required to become a trainer involves hard work and

application. Any doctor who does not have an interest in teaching should not become involved in vocational training.

2    Inevitably patients will have to see the trainee sometimes when they would have preferred to see their own doctor. In addition the inexperience of the trainee may result in misunderstandings with patients or, rarely, inappropriate and dangerous mistakes in management. The trainer will have to be very sensitive to this issue.

3    A good trainer will commit more of his/her time to the trainee than can be compensated for by shared workload in the practice. There will be tutorial times and acute situations where the trainer will find it impossible to just confine the time involved to previously agreed parameters. Lunchtimes will be eroded and trainers' workshops attended, often in the evenings. In addition several days a year will have to be set aside for special educational activities organized in the region.

## PREPARATION FOR TRAINING

### The trainer

A GP cannot become a trainer until he or she has been an established principal for at least 3–5 years. In addition to the experience required in clinical terms a prospective trainer will have to attend a trainers' course to learn about educational techniques and skills. In the south west region this requirement is a 1 week course before starting training and then a minimum of attendance at a 2-day seminar once every 3 years.

Trainers' workshops at a local level are important and occur for up to 2 hours every 2–4 weeks.

Within the practice adequate tutorial time will be required and joint surgeries with the trainee will normally be held once a week. The trainee will need to have their appointments carefully monitored so that they are not overloaded, especially in their early training. These implications for the appointment system will have to be discussed with the staff who will also have to be guided in the best way to introduce the trainee to the patients. The further implications to the practice of undertaking training activities are outlined below.

### The training practice

To be approved as a training practice quite a lot of preparatory work has to be undertaken and the responsibility for co-ordinating this will lie with the practice manager.

1   The records. Patient records must be of a high standard, with legible entries and a summary insert, in addition to being tidy and in order. Most of the systems outlined in the chapter on 'Records' must be available, such as a disease register and an age/sex register.

2   The building. The practice premises must be adequate for the number of partners and patients using them. It is preferable for the trainee to have his/her own room but if this is impossible then the timetable will have to be such that the trainee will be able to consult at his/her own rate without feeling under pressure to complete a surgery because someone else wishes to use the room. It is difficult to envisage practices without a treatment room being approved as the use of practice nurses within the surgery is now commonplace. It goes without saying that the overall impression must be welcoming, with clean premises in good repair.

3   The staff. The trainee should spend time in the reception area, waiting room, treatment room and with any other attached staff early in training so that he/she understands their role and gets to know them. The staff themselves should be familiar with the requirements of GP training with regard to their role. This will be particularly important for receptionists who will have the responsibility of making the appointments, controlling the trainee's workload and informing patients that they will be seeing a new doctor. The staff are also a good barometer of how well a trainee settles into the practice as they will soon get feedback from patients and form their own opinion. It is important for the practice manager to monitor this process as it may give an early warning of problems which the trainer will have to address with the trainee.

4   Timetable. Mention has already been made that the trainee will need to consult at a slower rate than the partners and the manager should discuss what the trainer and trainee wish in this respect. Protected teaching time for tutorials and joint surgeries is most important and the staff should understand the need for this arrangement and respect it.

5   Equipment. A training practice will have a great deal of equipment, from ECG machines to computers, and the manager must be certain that the trainee is given appropriate advice and training where necessary. The use of the computer is an example where the trainee will probably have had little experience of its use and the manager will have to arrange for instruction. Increasingly practices have their own video equipment for recording consultations and teaching sessions. The practice manager will have to be familiar with this equipment, be responsible for its security and liaise with the trainer on its use.

6   Practice library. Training practices are expected to have an adequate reference library for both the trainee and partners. Many practices set aside a specific sum of money each year to keep the library up to date and a partner is usually responsible for purchasing the books and journals. The manager will be responsible for ensuring the correct use of the library and establishing some system which will keep a check on the books. It is very easy for books to disappear as many people just 'borrow' them for a day or so and then forget to return them. Keeping some check on this will reduce the overheads of running the library.

7   Role in training. Practice managers should not underestimate their value in the training programme. Most doctors have few management skills and the trainee will probably be completely unfamiliar with management principles. As already described the manager will play an important part in establishing the trainee in the practice and this early relationship should be continued. During the year trainees have to learn as much as possible about practice management in preparation for joining their own practices and the manager will play a vital role in furthering this knowledge.

## CRITERIA FOR TRAINING PRACTICES

An outline has been given of the way that a practice will have prepared itself for training. Many regions now have formalized criteria which are used to measure the standards of the practice. In the south west region these come under a number of headings, for example:

1   The trainer as a clinician.
2   The trainer as a teacher.
3   The trainer as a member of the community.

Each criterion has a minimum standard, an average for the region, and good ideas introduced by a few practices. Criteria and standards do change from time to time and the trainer must keep the manager informed of the current standards. Practices will be reviewed using the criteria every 3–5 years depending on the regional arrangements.

## THE ASSESSMENT VISIT

It will now be clear that it takes some time for a practice and prospective GP trainer to prepare themselves to become a training practice. An application to be a trainer is submitted to the regional adviser in general practice once the prospective trainer is satisfied with his/her preparations. Following the application a visit may be made to the practice by the local course organizer of the GP Vocational

Training Scheme (VTS). This often happens if the applicant is from a new practice and the visit is intended to be supportive to the applicant and see if there are any obvious deficiencies which need to be amended before the formal visit.

The formal visit is either led by the regional adviser or his representative and includes a local course organizer and a course organizer or experienced trainer outside the local area. Details vary a little from region to region but the principles remain the same.

The aim of the visit is to assess the standard of the practice using the regional criteria and to check that the prospective trainer is adequately prepared for the role. It is intended that the tone of the visit should be friendly and educational and not punative. The visitors often wish to spend a brief time with the other partners to make sure that the trainer is supported in his/her application and will tour the premises paying particular attention to the record systems. After this they will discuss in detail with the trainer his/her plans and teaching strategies for the trainee.

The overall visit takes about 2 hours and, of course, during that time the trainer must be free and completely uninterrupted.

A revisit for renewal of an application after a GP has been a trainer already is somewhat different. The inspection of the premises is likely to be shorter although the record systems, appointment book and timetable will get some attention. More time will be spent in discussion with the trainer and the trainee (if in post at the time). It is becoming the norm in the south west region for a trainer to show a video recording of a tutorial. This is discussed with the visitors constructively so that the trainer may continue to improve his/her skills.

The manager's responsibility will be to greet the visitors, make sure that arrangements go smoothly and answer any questions which might be asked of them about the organizational side of the practice.

It should be emphasized that if a training practice is enthusiastic and well prepared the visit should be a pleasurable event with an opportunity for the practice to benefit from the opinions of impartial outside observers. No matter how good a practice is there are always opportunities for new ideas to be introduced.

## THE TRAINING ENVIRONMENT

The manager will not be involved in training outside the practice unless invited to participate in a local teaching session. However it is important to understand where the practice fits into the local GP training environment.

An outline of the organizational responsibility for training is shown in Figure 10.1.

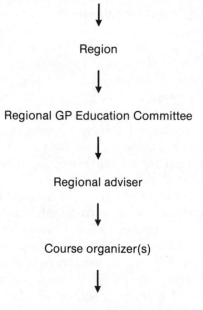

Joint Committee on Postgraduate Training for General Practice

Region

Regional GP Education Committee

Regional adviser

Course organizer(s)

Training practice

**Fig. 10.1**    Organizational responsibility for training.

All trainers will be associated with a local VTS. This will be organized by one or more course organizers who are responsible for the co-ordination of GP training in the area. They will organize a half day release course for all trainees in their area and each training practice will be expected to incorporate the trainee's attendance at this course into their timetable. Many doctors on a VTS have an introductory period of 1–3 months in general practice and then complete 2 years in a hospital post before returning to general practice to complete their training. Practices may be involved with the first or last of these attachments or both. A practice may also take a trainee for 1 complete year if they have already done their hospital posts.

The regional adviser is the executive officer of the Regional GP Education Committee which is responsible for all GP training in the region. His role will be to co-ordinate training activities in the region and liaise with the course organizers. He will be responsible for dealing with any training problems which occur and trainers are encouraged to liaise closely with him and the local course organizer(s).

The overall regulatory body for GP training nationally is the Joint Committee on Postgraduate Training for General Practice (JCPTGP). For most practices this will be a remote body but it is responsible for giving formal approval to a trainee at the end of training before entering practice as a principal.

In addition they are responsible for an occasional visit to the region to monitor standards and as part of this regional assessment a training practice may find itself visited by the representatives of the JCPTGP. If this does occur the regional adviser and local course organizer will liaise with the practice and give them guidelines but in general terms it is no different from an assessment visit to be a trainer.

## APPOINTMENT OF A TRAINEE

Under the terms and conditions of service (the Red Book) the trainer is responsible for employing the trainee even if they have been appointed through the local VTS.

As with any other practice appointment the prospective trainee will have to be interviewed and approved. The manager may be responsible for advertising the vacancy through the medical journals and making arrangements for interested applicants to visit the practice.

Once appointed the trainee will have a contract like any other employee. In addition to the normal contract of employment there is a contract related to training and trainers are encouraged to get their trainees to sign this too.

The trainee is paid via the FHSA, who will refund the salary to the practice, but the manager will be responsible for administering this and making sure that PAYE and NI contributions are deducted. The trainee also gets a car allowance. Discussions will have to take place between the local tax office and the practice as to whether the allowance can be paid as an expense or whether it should be taxed and the trainee claim this back later. The situation varies from place to place.

There are also many other allowances to which trainees may be entitled, such as the installation of a telephone at home. The manager should be familiar with these which are all detailed in the Red Book. If in doubt the trainee should discuss the problem with the FSHA or local course organizer.

There are many rewards in becoming a training practice despite the hard work in preparation for it. The practice manager will play a key role in this development.

## FURTHER READING

*Recommendations to Regions for the Establishment of Criteria for the Approval and Reapproval of Trainers in General Practice.* Joint Committee on Postgraduate Training for General Practice, 14 Princes Gate, Hyde Park, London, 1985.

Gray Pereira D.J. (1982) *Training for General Practice*. Macdonald and Evans, 1982.

Hall M.S. (1989) *A GP Training Handbook*, second edition. Blackwell Scientific Publications, Oxford.

# Chapter 11

# Training for Practice Staff

Until recently there have been very few formal training courses for staff, whether they be practice managers, practice nurses or receptionists. Most that have been available have either been short study days or part of training for a specific qualification such as medical secretary.

However, during the last few years matters have changed dramatically as the needs of practice staff have begun to be recognized by doctors and by a variety of providers.

By the end of the chapter you should:

1 Be aware of the training needs of staff.
2 Be aware of the variety of opportunities available to meet these needs.

The 1990 contract has given a great boost to this training boom as part of the contract is that staff should be provided with adequate opportunities to train. Indeed FHSAs now have money available for practices for training purposes. Some FHSAs are giving practices their own training budget to use on staff training needs as they see fit. There is no doubt that this boom will continue and that within a short time all staff will expect to have training opportunities on an annual basis.

The decision as to whom should have training and what, depending on the facilities available, will be the responsibility of the practice manager in discussion with the partners.

## IN SERVICE TRAINING

It has been traditional for the majority of practice staff to be trained by exposure to the job and learning by total immersion! Unfortunately, while this type of learning may be valuable, some people inevitably drown!

In-service training can be used for reception and nursing staff and, indeed, to some extent no amount of training will prepare a receptionist for the stresses of a busy Monday morning in winter until she has been in post and gained confidence and experience.

In-service training of the staff must be planned carefully by the practice manager so that a new member of staff is sequentially introduced to her tasks and, ideally, she should be seen to be proficient at one before passing on to the next. This is rarely possible but a number of guidelines might help to lessen the stress of introducing a new member of staff to her role. Informal training should commence on the first day of work.

1   Prepare an induction programme, planning a timetable from the first day of employment. Include time with as many members of the practice and primary health care team as possible, to give a general idea of roles and responsibilities.
2   Inform all members of the team of the name, role and starting time and date of the new member of staff and of the time and date that they will be expected to look after them. Ask them to wear name badges. Even in a small practice it is often difficult to remember names immediately.
3   Welcome the new person and introduce them to people as soon as is practicable. Show them round the surgery again, even if they had a tour at interview. They are likely to have forgotten the layout.
4   Give full information on fire and health and safety regulations.
5   Go through the job description discussing various aspects of the job. These will be written in the contract but more detail or clarification will be required. This will be an appropriate time to emphasize the confidential aspects of her work.
6   Decide on the ranking order for learning the different aspects of the job.
7   Ideally the initial induction period should last about 2 weeks. During this time periods spent with the members of the team, such as the practice nurse, the district nurse, the health visitor, and various members of the reception and administrative staff, will give a sound basis on which future training can be built.
8   Progress from this to a graded timetable in which all aspects of the role are introduced in turn. The explanation of various tasks will probably be best carried out by the member of staff most proficient in that area. It is not always necessary for the practice manager to spend a lot of time training personally. However, it is important to monitor progress regularly. One way of doing this is for the member of staff to rate their own performance for each specific task and then for the manager to rate it. If there is any discrepancy in the marking it gives a basis for discussion as to why the member

of staff rates themselves higher, or lower, than the manager, and can identify the need for further training or practice.

9  The new member of staff should gradually assume responsibility as her/his experience increases. During this time the practice manager will have to be sensitive to feedback from partners, patients and other members of the team about performance. Observation of how the telephone is answered, or a patient is dealt with at the reception desk, will be useful.

In-service training for practice nurses is also common and the same principles apply, although the actual training will be the responsibility of the senior practice nurse. Basic training courses for practice nurses are almost obligatory now and this will be discussed later.

Other members of staff will need training, which can be in house, if they have a specific skill to learn. These would include computer users, filing clerks, dispensers or nurse aides.

Appraisal of staff gives an excellent opportunity to identify the training needs of existing staff. Ideally each member of staff should complete a questionnaire which asks them to identify their strengths and weaknesses, and how they feel that they can be helped to overcome their weaknesses and develop their strengths. Ample, uninterrupted, time should be set aside for full discussion. It may be possible to identify hidden skills, or for the person to express their ambitions. For the manager it will also help in planning for the future if the full range of skills of the staff is known.

Once having identified areas where help is needed it is possible to plan the best method of learning for the individual concerned. This may be by in-house training, but it could also be by finding suitable external training or reading material. External training may mean going on a course, but it could also involve distance learning.

Full use should be made of the training skills of the whole team, including the doctors, when arranging in-house training. Some of this may be on a one to one basis but group sessions can also be effective. In a medium to large surgery it is cost effective to contract with external experts to provide, say, an evening on telephone skills, or on assertiveness. Visits to the FHSA, and the local hospital pathology laboratory, X-ray department and ambulance control offer insight into how other organizations work. This can be beneficial to both parties leading to greater understanding.

Training can be an excellent motivating factor in the practice team. It should be accepted that we need to continue to develop our knowledge and skills throughout our working life.

## SPECIAL TRAINING COURSES

### Receptionists

Many organizations, from night schools to polytechnics, are now offering some form of receptionist training. The quality of this will vary and the practice manager should satisfy himself or herself that the course being offered is appropriate to the training needs of the member of staff concerned. The more the providers are familiar with the staff roles in general practice the more likely the course is to be appropriate. For example, if the course is organized by a general practitioner or practice manager it is far more likely to be of relevance than one organized by a polytechnic tutor.

Radcliffe Medical Press have developed a training package for receptionists – PRP – which is being used throughout the country. This package is useful but expensive and unlikely to meet anything other than a basic need as it is not flexible.

The Association of Medical Secretaries, Practice Administrators and Receptionists (AMSPAR) also offers courses.

### Practice nurses

As the role of the practice nurse has developed in the last decade a need for a basic training course has been recognized. Some of the early courses, such as those organized in the Department of General Practice at Exeter, were the results of initiatives of various individuals, but training is now becoming more formalized. The English Nursing Board (ENB) is responsible for approving courses for nurses and it is very likely that as time goes by most of the basic training courses will be ENB approved. Allied to the basic training will probably be some form of practice attachment to a nurse trainer under a system similar to the GP training programme. However, the funding and timing of this type of course is still a long way from being decided.

In the past few years specific training courses for practice nurses in their extended role have developed. The most well known example of these is the Asthma Training Centre in Stratford where many nurses have developed skills in assessing and managing asthmatic patients. This is a highly popular course and a trainers programme has also been developed for those interested in teaching these skills to other nurses.

Study days and an annual national conference are now organized throughout the country.

The Department of General Practice in Exeter has developed the philosophy of multidisciplinary training and since 1989 has offered a joint GP/PN trainers course to meet the new training needs of those practice nurses who will become trainers. There are also opportunities for the taking of a higher degree, for example an MSc or other specialist qualification.

## Practice managers

Practice managers now have a great many training opportunities to improve their skills.

There are a variety of business management courses available either locally through further education sources or via the Open University. Certainly a practice manager who has reached his or her position in practice through long service and without formal training should now insist on this type of training course.

The AHCPA has designed and developed a structured programme which is nationally recognized and is suitable for a range of people, from those aspiring to be managers, working within practice or outside, to the general manager who has responsibility for the overall control of the practice and the fund holding manager. This training is provided via a network of people working in regions that correspond to the Regional Health Authority areas. Each of these areas has a representative, the Regional Education Administrator (REA), who is a member of the national education team and is the contact person for managers enquiring about training.

These people work with colleges, polytechnics and universities who also run AHCPA courses. The national team plans and develops the education programme, monitors standards and evaluates the training courses. All members of the team are practising practice managers, members of the Association, take part in regular 'training for trainers' courses and undergo performance review. They meet regularly at a regional and a national level.

The content of the programme is modularized and there is flexibility in its provision that allows regions to respond to local needs. The foundation module is an introduction to practice management which covers basic finance, employment and health and safety laws, the roles of the practice manager and the FHSA, and systems and communications. The four modules at the intermediate level are: managing people, managing money, managing information and resources, and communicating effectively. The advanced level has three modules: performance review, training for trainers, and leadership for managers.

The assessment for the new AHCPA Diploma comprises: a multiple choice questionnaire, an essay, in-house evidence of competence, and preparing and presenting a project. Accreditation will come from BTec, endorsement from the Management Charter Initiative, and a

Certificate in Management Studies will be awarded. Prior learning is accredited on an individual basis, thus allowing suitably qualified people exemption from certain modules, although some may have to produce evidence of competence.

The Association's initiative with the Open University led to the adaptation of some of the material of the 'Managing Health Services' module for general practice, and other courses comprising the Professional Certificate and Diploma in Management and the MBA programme being offered at a discount.

The AHCPA will continue to develop their training programme to respond to national and local needs. Currently, with the advent of national vocational qualifications, it is ensuring that courses are compatible with the requirements of the scheme.

The AMSPAR, who represent all practice administrative staff, also have a programme of courses which cater for receptionists, secretaries, administrators and managers. This too culminates in a diploma, for practice administration. Their programme enables people to take a series of courses to progress and obtain promotion within practice and are provided through colleges of further information.

The MSc courses mentioned earlier for practice nurses are also available in some areas of the country for managers too.

Elsewhere in this book (Chapter 10) mention has been made of the importance of training and the fact that it will not be long before all members of the team expect to have the same amount of formal study leave or training as doctors. It will be the responsibility of the manager to co-ordinate all these activities and see that appropriate opportunities are offered to all staff.

For further information contact:

The Education Co-ordinator, AHCPA, c/o 14 Princes Gate, Hyde Park, London SW1 7PU.

The Secretary, AMSPAR, Tavistock House North, Tavistock Square, London.

The Department of General Practice, Postgraduate Medical School, Barrack Road, Exeter.

# Chapter 12

# General Principles of Management

## INTRODUCTION AND OBJECTIVES

Practice management is a new business. In a time of rapid change and introduction of managerial ideas new to primary care, managers rightly require a set of principles that can be used to make effective decisions. These principles, however, are not universal, but are generalizations that have arisen from experiences in various organizations.

The term 'management' has been defined in a variety of ways. Each definition has several key components. The first of these is planning. Management is about thinking of the future, about having a dream of the direction in which the practice should be striving. The second is about present effectiveness, about having the systems, personnel and strategies available to enable the smooth and efficient running of the practice today. The third is about personal effectiveness, about time management, people-centred skills and good communication skills.

These components combine to give a broad view of management in primary health care – the ability to redirect and focus the skills and potential of today's team into the future. Handy (1985) describes these as the concepts that help one to explain the past, allow one to understand the present and to predict the future. This gives greater influence over future events and thus less disturbance from the unexpected. This requires some understanding and analysis of the core principles of management.

At the end of this chapter you should:

1  Have an outline knowledge of the history of management theories.
2  Have an understanding of the major principles involved in managing a practice.
3  Be able to apply these principles to the everyday running of your practice.

## HISTORY OF MANAGEMENT THEORY

Managerial ideas have their roots in ancient history, for example with the building of the pyramids. Machiavelli, in the sixteenth century, developed principles based on mass consent, leadership, cohesiveness and the will to survive. With the industrial revolution and development of factories, scientific management arose, consisting of ideas such as forecasting quality, control and work studies. Taylor in 1912, in his *Principles of Scientific Management* laid down some of the foundations of modern management, basing his principles on the reduction of observation to laws and rules. Fayol, a French mining engineer, was the first to construct a complete theory of management in 1916, in which he divided management activities into five elements: planning, organizing, directing, co-ordinating and controlling.

Mayo in 1933 was the first to research extensively into management activities; his study on motivation at the Hawthorne electrical works remains a classic (Mayo 1949). Traditional management principles lost favour after the war for a variety of reasons, not the least being a lack of empirical research. To some degree this has been redressed with the work of Maslow into the hierarchical system of individual motivation (Maslow 1954) and studies by Herzberg of 'hygiene' factors at work (Herzberg 1966). More recently, researchers have concentrated on the structure and effectiveness of organizations and on operational research.

The ideas that came from these writers are many. Key terms include:

1  Systems.
2  Balance.
3  Innovation.
4  Delegation.
5  Leadership.
6  Flexibility.

### Systems:

Organizations consist of a wide range of activities interconnected to form systems. Deciding on who or what is part of a system is an important aspect of management.

### Balance:

An organization is a balance between the demands and constraints of those outside it and the needs of those inside it. For example, the desire for patients to have appointments at unsocial times, against which has to be set the needs of staff for proper leisure time.

### Innovation:

Forward planning is a vital part of effective management. An important aspect of this is not only having the ability to think up new ideas, but also being aware of creativity in others and fostering rather than hindering this process. This involves creating and nurturing a climate conducive to innovation.

### Delegation:

This includes not only deciding which tasks are suitable for delegation, but also developing systems for motivating and monitoring staff.

### Leadership:

Whether leadership qualities are innate or skills which may be learnt is debatable. But what does seem clear is that the effective manager has the ability to take decisions, has integrity, enthusiasm, imagination, and is prepared to work hard. *Esprit de corps* was one key idea in Fayol's principles of management (Fayol 1916).

### Flexibility:

Changing situations demand the ability to adapt. There is a need to be sensitive to the needs of others both inside and outside the system. A sense of humour and perspective are valuable elements of the skilled manager.

## CURRENT THEORIES OF MANAGEMENT

Space prevents a detailed analysis of all aspects of management skills. The six most important issues will be discussed here:

1  Planning.
2  The management of change.
3  Issues of leadership.
4  Motivation.
5  Monitoring.
6  Time management.

## Planning

Every manager has a plan. It means thinking about the unexpected and having systems to deal with it. An example of this in primary care would be the effect on the practice of a new housing development that might cause an influx of patients onto the list. The effective manager who has planned will have considered both the implications of this change on the workload of the practice and over what period it would be likely to take place.

Sudden and rapid changes in society and health care force the practice manager to carry out planning strategies in order for the primary health care team (PHCT) to function. Examples of these changes include information technology and the growth in patient demand.

The process of planning consists of four stages:

1   Setting objectives.
2   Collecting information related to these objectives.
3   Examining and evaluating courses of action.
4   Selecting, recommending and carrying out the chosen course.

### Setting objectives

Objectives can be global or specific. Global objectives are those where the team sets the overall aim of the practice. This is the mission or corporate statement of a practice, which should be stated in terms that are appropriate to the particular locality. It would be too wide to set an aim of being the best practice in the UK, but more realistic to have the aim of providing high quality care to a particular locality.

Specific objectives should be precise and measurable. This measurement can be either quantitative or qualitative. For example, a practice may set the objective of moving from 8 minute to 10 minute appointments by the end of the financial year. Whether this has been done or not is quantitative and easily measured. A qualitative measurement would be, for example, to see whether patients are satisfied by a particular course of action in the practice such as a non-appointment surgery. The measurement here is less precise, but no less important and valuable.

A practice may well have multiple objectives. Setting too many goals to achieve in a short time can be stressful, so it is helpful to set some priorities for these, regarding when they should be achieved, how and by whom.

The difficulty of translating traditional business management experience to primary care is that practices do not exist wholly to make a profit. This can in part be overcome by thinking of value in the service offered to patients. Some of the ideas espoused by Drucker can be transposed to general practice (Drucker 1955). In business terms, he suggests the following should be key objectives for a company:

1 Profitability.
2 Market position.
3 Productivity.
4 Product leadership.
5 Personal development.
6 Employee attitudes.
7 Public responsibility.
8 Balance between short and long term objectives.

*Profitability:* In primary care, instead of profitability being an objective, value to the patient and society can be considered. An example of value here might be ensuring child immunization uptake rates are acceptable, both from an individual child's point of view and for the general population in that area.

*Market position:* This is related to the population demands the practice is attempting to meet. For example, the siting of the surgery, the number of partners or the appointment hours offered depend on the population the PHCT serves.

*Productivity:* A throughput objective would be to analyse the number of patients seen in a certain length of time.

*Product leadership:* This says something about the quality of care offered to those on the list (see chapter on Audit).

*Public responsibility:* This has always been the concern of general practice. Beyond clinical responsibilities, many health care workers give their time to voluntary bodies, but with current restraints the time devoted to these may have to be reconsidered.

*Personal development:* This is for each individual within the PHCT. It aims to help the person work at their highest possible level and in a way most satisfying to them.

*Employee attitudes:* This includes the ethos and global objectives of the team and each individual's contribution to fulfilling them. In general practice terms, the idea is best used by looking at the attitudes of those working in the team, whether they are partners or staff.

*Balance:* This must always be set between short and long term objectives. Excessive concentration on the short term fails to look at the overall future for the practice. Looking solely at long term objectives fails to take account of targets which must be met to achieve the overall aim. Long term goals may appear at first impossible to meet. Short term objectives motivate PHCT members to meet these long term goals.

As outside demands change, so objectives need to change with them. Certainly, appraisal of objectives, particularly long term ones, needs to be built into planning. Some practices use a system of both 5-year and 1-year plans. Each year, the 1-year plan is adjusted to take account of changes that have occurred both within the organization and externally. This is incorporated within, and reflects, the 5-year plan.

To achieve objectives, they must be transmitted to all members of the team. Failure to do so usually results in under achievement and demoralization. Objectives are more likely to be met if all members of a team are part of the planning process itself. They then own the objectives rather than having them imposed from above. Planning meetings involving all members of the team help achieve this. Ownership of the objectives enables individuals to make the best use of their skills and the resources available to them.

### Collecting information

Data gathering is time consuming, but without all relevant information decisions taken may not be the best. This requires the practice manager to delegate effectively. To do this, a knowledge of the skill mix of the team and the workload of each individual is needed. Despite this, information will probably never be complete, and there has to be a balance between waiting until all relevant data are collected, when deadlines may be missed, and acting without having all the facts.

### Examining and evaluation

Management involves decision making, which necessarily implies a choice between more than one action. Part of planning is to examine these alternatives and evaluate which options might be preferable. It is important to select criteria before taking a decision, such as whether to lease or to buy a computer system. The practice will have to set criteria against which they can judge the decision, such as how they want to use their capital.

### Selecting, recommending and implementing

Decision making is often quoted as a key managerial activity. Space precludes a detailed look at the theory of decision making here. One example of a suggested approach is to list objectives and put them in priority order. This enables one to see which decision will produce the desired outcome.

Recommending the selected course of action is another key task of managers. This will involve considering who is to deliver the recommendations and the recipients. Timing is always crucial to managerial activity, no less so than deciding when to make the recommendation. Consideration must be given to how the ideas are communicated. In general practice, it may be hard for the partners to accept recommendations from junior staff. With thought, the manager can ensure that the ideas are received appropriately.

It is often likely that those carrying out the decisions will not be the same members of the team as the planners. It is possible that implementers may feel discomfort at having to put into effect a plan conceived by someone else. One solution to this potential area of conflict is to ensure that the implementers have an awareness of and, if possible, contribute to the planning process. This also often solves many practical problems before they arise. Receptionists may point out glaring faults in a proposed appointment system that others cannot see.

In order for all to be involved, it is helpful to examine the practical issues and the belief systems in which people operate. For example, a late health promotion clinic may suit the patients. However, the work routine of the cleaner may be inconvenienced. Consultation and negotiation need to occur at the planning stage.

Plans are static, but events outside are dynamic. Since planning takes time, it is crucial to find out that the decisions are still applicable. It may be necessary to fine tune the planning process to meet the continually changing needs of the practice.

## The management of change

Life is change. We develop. External circumstances alter. In response to new situations we change our perception of the world.

Despite this, we tend to resist change. We are inclined to see it in terms of difficulties and obstacles rather than opportunities and challenges. There are probably many reasons for this. They may include our culture, our previous education, our life experience and our personality. Individuals tend to be attached to their roots, social and organizational as well as geographical. Change may involve a severance of these attachments that could affect personal well-being.

Organizations and individuals react to change emotionally rather than logically. Rational argument may lead to entrenchment rather than co-operation. Strategies must be used that ease the transition for people. This transition needs to be consciously managed. Consideration should be given to the rate of change, to how much change really needs to take place, and to the commitment of those involved. A review process evaluating the system after the change must be in place.

It is helpful to differentiate between transition (which is possible) and transformation (which is difficult). Change involving transition should be aimed at rather than expecting a complete transformation. With any change, there will be gainers and losers. Consideration must be given to those who feel they are losing; they must feel compensated in some way. The overall effect will then be a net gain to the welfare of the practice.

There are several useful strategies that simplify change:

1  Force field analysis.
2  Zooming.
3  Reframing.
4  Handling conflict.
5  Identifying key personnel.

### Force field analysis

This is a technique that is described in detail elsewhere (Lewin 1951). The essence is to:

1  Define the problem in specific terms.
2  Identify who is involved and their systems.
3  Decide the size of the problem.
4  List any other factors involved.
5  Decide clearly on the target so you know when it is reached.
6  List the forces operating on the problem: identify pushing forces – those which move the present situation towards the goal; and identify restraining forces – those which resist movement towards the goal.
7  Detect new pushing forces, while reducing restraining forces.
8  Divert restraining forces elsewhere.
9  Remember that it may be possible for an apparently pushing force to act as a restraining force (for example, personal eagerness to effect the change).

### Zooming

This consists of firstly examining the roots of a problem by asking 'why?' An example would be the problem of requests to arrange more meetings. The technique is to ask why meetings are necessary – perhaps for communication. Why is there a need to communicate through meetings? The problem has now been redefined. The second stage is to zoom in to this new problem. There are many methods of communicating. Meetings provide only one medium. We could write, phone or delegate the decision making. These may not be answers to this situation, but by stepping back, and then zooming in, we have looked at the problem in a new way.

## Reframing

This follows on from the previous suggestion. We may be able to turn problems into opportunities by removing previously understood boundaries, taking a new look at what exists. This may arise from zooming, but can also arise by deliberately resetting boundaries. A member of staff who is continually questioning practice could be looked on as a creative thinker.

## Handling conflict

Many people often avoid conflict because it seems destructive. Conflict reflects energy, energy that could be harnessed to help change. People who resist change may be as committed to the planned outcome as you, but may disagree on the method of change. By understanding them as individuals, appreciating their concerns and criticisms, it is possible that resistance to change may be overcome.

## Identifying key personnel

The types of individuals found in teams have been described elsewhere in this book. Many will be allies in helping you effect change. The organizer is the person who will drive the change through. The team worker will check that team members are not being damaged through the change. In every team there is one who is the opinion leader, the person who is credible, and who is able to persuade the team that a certain change is good. Identify this person, explain the change fully and the benefits which would result. As an ally, they will be valuable in supporting your objective. The most effective change is one owned by all, and therefore the initiator or innovator may not get the credit. One hard aspect of being a manager and leader is that credit may not be given where it actually belongs. A leader has to accept that it is the change that is important, not the person who led it.

## Issues of leadership

Few would doubt that leaders exist, but the criteria of leadership are harder to define. Theories abound as to why some are 'better' leaders than others. For a time, it was felt that leaders were born, not made;

leadership was an inborn trait that people either possessed or did not. This view has largely been discredited, and more in favour is the notion that individuals have certain qualities that empower them to take the leadership role.

Examples of these qualities are the ability to take decisions, the ability to work both hard and long hours, integrity, enthusiasm, imagination and people-centred skills. Some of these seem innate, but clearly others are skills and can be learnt. Leadership is a blend of the current situation, the qualities of the leader, and the characteristics of the group being led. In many situations it is appropriate for the situation to decide on who should be leader. This raises the issue that leaders are leaders in some situations but not others. What does seem important is that given the right situation, integrity (trust and truth), enthusiasm, warmth, calmness and a sense of being tough but fair, are all important. The group gives credibility to someone who reflects the group norms, but who is seen to be slightly more able than the group members.

Autocratic and democratic leadership illustrate two contrasting notions. Autocratic leaders tend to be dictatorial and paternalistic. They achieve goals by orders and threats rather than by involvement. On the other hand, democratic leaders reach goals by consultative and participative methods. The latter runs the risk of lacking a positive direction, but promotes morale and stimulates initiative. Leaders need to promote creativity and problem solving in teams. Autocracy tends to stifle this, whereas democracy advances it. Clearly, there are situations where autocracy is necessary. The approach is to think carefully about which decisions require consultation and which do not.

A key feature of leaders appears to be their perception and sensitivity to a situation, with an appropriate response. They also have the ability to motivate others. They have the particular capacity of being able to stand back from a problem, review all elements, identify the solutions, and then to communicate this vision to the rest of the team.

To end, the manner in which an individual operates in a particular situation reflects their leadership capability. It should be borne in mind that leadership requires a person to build on experience, not repeat it.

## Motivation

As mentioned previously, leaders have the ability to motivate staff. Maslow studied motivation factors and prioritized these into physiology, safety, sociability, self-esteem, and self-actualization (Maslow 1954). Lower levels must first be satisfied before an individual can operate at the higher levels. So, for example, staff will not work efficiently if they are cold or hungry. Also, staff will find difficulty in using their own initiative if they are not valued as people.

Individuals will only be motivated to achieve the goal if they perceive the worth and value of the task, and that it is congruent with their values and beliefs. Boring or tedious work still needs to be done. In this case it helps to identify people who feel least affected by the routine or who have a particular skill that is harnessed. For these tasks, a financial reward may be more appropriate than depending on a sense of achievement.

McGregor identified two styles of management, calling them theory X and theory Y (McGregor 1960). A theory X manager believes that people avoid work if possible. Workers need inducements and sanctions and are reluctant to assume responsibility, preferring defined tasks rather than broad objectives. In contrast to this, a theory Y manager believes that people will work hard without coercion. They can be relied on for self-direction, and actively seek out responsibility. They have potential that needs developing.

Herzberg distinguished motivating factors from hygiene factors (Herzberg 1966). Motivators are factors such as achievement and recognition, whereas hygiene factors do not, in themselves, motivate but, if absent, will cause dissatisfaction. His work suggests that motivators are not aspects such as pay and conditions, but are, for example, job satisfaction and responsibility.

## Monitoring

Managers not only plan and implement, they also monitor. They assess what is going on, evaluate a course of action and change, and feedback on performance. Feedback is important to morale. As we have seen from Maslow's work, people need to know when they have done well, and need recognition for achievement. To be effective, feedback needs to be as soon after the performance as possible.

Poor results or mistakes also need to be pointed out as soon as they become apparent. Delay in discussing where someone is going wrong for fear of hurting their feelings will only cause anger and resentment and will reduce its potency as a learning tool. This type of feedback requires a combination of messages. Firstly that the person is valued by you, and secondly a clear statement on the aspect of behaviour that is causing concern. Separating your feelings for them as a person and the behaviour is crucial when giving negative feedback.

In planning a new initiative, a manager must identify the intended outcome and how that can be proven to have occurred. Some forms of evaluation consider whether the outcome is effective, efficient and whether the cost to the practice has been justified. It is also critical to identify forms of evaluation that examine the quality of care given to, and satisfaction of, the patient.

## Time management

Time is a precious resource, yet many of us manage it less effectively than any other aspects of our work. Effective managers show the ability to structure their personal time. This seems to include time that is available when needed for other people. There are many manuals and books on time management, so only an outline of some of the strategies that can be studied is made here.

Adair (1987) lists key points as:

1   Time is money: cost out the tasks of the day.
2   Check out how you actually use the time in the day.
3   Common problems are procrastination; failure to delegate; lack of efficiency in the office; unnecessary meetings; and failure to identify priorities.
4   Identify long term goals.
5   Make middle term plans.
6   Plan your use of time for the day.
7   Identify your own quality time and use it effectively.
8   Organize your office.
9   Handle papers only once.
10  Control interruptions – 'I've got 5 minutes'.
11  Manage meetings effectively – are they really necessary?
12  Delegate, don't do.
13  Make use of committed time (for example on journeys).
14  Take care of your health and relaxation needs.

## CONCLUSION

In general practice, leadership comes from many members of the team. A manager in general practice has to balance the resources of a team with the demands of the patient group and society. Team commitment to an effective and efficient management of resources, including people, results in quality health care. Management tasks within the PHCT may be shared amongst many members, but it is important for one person to retain a view of the team as a whole and the direction in which it is moving. This allows planning, whilst building on the experiences of the past.

## REFERENCES

Adair J. (1987) *How to Manage your Time*. Talbot Adair.

Drucker P. (1955) *The Practice of Management*. Pan Books.

Fayol H. (1916) Quoted in *General and Industrial Management*, Pitman, 1949, translated by Constance Storrs.

Handy C.B. (1985) In *Understanding Organisations*, Penguin Books, Harmondsworth.

Herzberg F. (1966) *Work and the Nature of the Man*. World Publishing Company.

Lewin K. (1951) *Field Theory in Social Science*. Harper.

Maslow A. (1954) *Motivation & Personality*. Harper & Row.

Mayo, E. (1949) *The Social Problems of an Industrial Civilisation*. Routledge.

McGregor D. (1960) *The Human Side of Enterprise*. McGraw-Hill.

Taylor F. (1912) Testimony to the House of Representatives Committee, quoted in *Scientific Management*, Harper & Row, 1947.

# Chapter 13

# Working in Teams

## INTRODUCTION AND OBJECTIVES

As primary care grows more and more complex, opportunities unfold for individual members of the team to deal with the varying situations that arise. It is essential that the whole team functions as one unit, each member using their expertise while recognizing the skills of other members. They have a common purpose, identifying themselves as members of a team and being acknowledged as such by others outside that group. Every person has characteristics, such as drive, enthusiasm and finishing skills, which if combined in one individual might be in conflict, yet in a group such variety can unite to give added strength. The ideal team consists of a group of individuals who between them have qualities of leadership, energy, innovation, social skills and finishing abilities.

This chapter will look at the variety of skills and approaches found in teams, the roles individuals can bring to a group and how to set about developing a successful team. At the end of the chapter you should:

1  Understand the nature of a team.
2  Understand the skills that individuals can bring to a team.
3  Understand the qualities of your own team.
4  Understand how to select new members for your team.

## THE NATURE OF TEAMS

For a team to be successful, it should ideally consist of people with differences rather than similarities. A football team with 11 goal-keepers would not be successful. Similarly, a primary care team that consisted entirely of innovators would be full of ideas but lacking action. The aim of a team is to achieve a common goal rather than reach a compromise situation. This common purpose contrasts with that of a committee, which is a collection of representatives who are attempting to find solutions acceptable to all. Teams are collections of individuals with loyalties to the team and a common purpose.

Becoming a member of a team has implications for each of us. Any new entrant goes through anxiety on joining, established members feel lost when they leave, and membership itself of the team imparts a sense of worth to its members. Teams as groups experience some of the worries that individuals have – such as anxiety on arrival of new members, and the need to accommodate them into its well established structure. Joining a new team requires us to redefine our roles and how we see ourselves, which may, in turn, affect our personal values. The achievements of the team as a whole affect each individual's self-esteem. For example, success in treating a patient can be valued by all, and a mistake will be experienced by all.

A factor common to all teams is the interdependence of members of that organization. Lewin suggests that cohesiveness occurs when individuals realize that their fate depends on the future of the team as a whole (Lewin 1948). External forces may amplify this. For example, the new contract helped many teams develop cohesion and unity.

Lewin suggests that the achievement of personal goals of individual members contributes to the development of the team (Lewin 1948). A team consisting of people with complementary skills, each of whom is successful, enables others in the team to achieve, so furthering the team goals. For example, a skilful receptionist can enhance clinical work. A competitive atmosphere will damage the overall performance of the organization. Competitive teams are doomed to show poor results.

Problems may arise that threaten the stability of the team. There may, for example, be a conflict in values between members, or outside pressure may produce different demands on individuals. Bales, in his study of group function, recognized these difficulties (Bales 1950). However, he believed that in general, threats tended to be positive or reinforcing rather than negative.

Bales also observed that groups went through phases in their development. Initially a group has to orient itself both to the individuals and to the task. After a period of orientation (forming), individuals in the group may show some competitive behaviour, attempting to control decision making (storming). Following this uneasy time, group norms may be set concerning behaviour, control and communication (norming). After this there is a period of good teamwork, with co-operation, collaboration and achievement of team aims (performing).

An example of this may be seen when a partner joins a practice. Initially individuals get to know each other and their working procedures. After a while, the partner suggests alterations to the structures and routine. Ideally those involved discuss the problem and various options, resulting in a team commitment to a solution. Failure to achieve this will result in chronic dissatisfaction of all concerned.

The norming phase defines the limits of acceptable and unacceptable behaviour. In a health care setting this may be concerned with dress, communication channels or other aspects of interpersonal behaviour, for example whether team members use each others' first names. Norms in behaviour are important in helping an individual to structure and predict what will happen in the team. They also have an important role in group cohesiveness. This will result in the team achieving its goals. Group norms tend to persist through several generations of team members.

## INDIVIDUALS AND TEAMS

Individuals bring both strengths and weaknesses to a team. Not only do they have skills and talents that make them suited to a task, they also have personal qualities which help or hinder the team's performance. Personality plays a part here, but personality cannot easily change. Some find it easy to socialize and enjoy a lot of contact with others, whilst some are loners. Some tend to control, whereas others prefer to be directed. Finally, there are those who easily form relationships, whereas some people are more wary of entering such associations. These aspects of personality have been explored by Schutz in the FIRO-B personality test (Schutz 1958). Teams need to adjust and adapt to these individual differences, both making allowances for them as well as seeing them as potential strengths.

Closely related to personality, but more amenable to change, are particular behavioural traits. Honey and Mumford usefully divided learning styles into four categories – activist, reflector, theorist and pragmatist (Honey & Mumford 1982). Though this work related to learning, it is useful to look at an individual's behaviour in these four terms.

Activists tend to take decisions rapidly without much thought. They tend to be impatient of those who are slower. The quality of an activist's decisions, because they are fast, may not always be sound. Reflectors, on the other hand, need time. They need to process information and consider it for perhaps several days before reaching a conclusion. They may need to talk to others or seek references before deciding on a course of action. This care usually results in a quality decision, but it does take time and time may not always be available.

Theorists prefer the notion of systems, the reasons why things happen, and logical deductive arguments. They may doggedly stick to a point of view, disrupting the natural flow of a meeting because they are sure they are right or have reason behind their argument. Nevertheless, their theoretical knowledge and persistence in challenging assumptions can be very useful in team meetings. Pragmatists tend to identify problems and solutions. They tend to be practically rather than theoretically oriented. Their strength in the team will be to identify and put into practice the team decisions, but they may opt for one solution rather than examining all possibilities.

Most people show a mixture of all four styles, with one or two dominating. Each style has its strengths and weaknesses. The key is to use the strengths of each individual for the benefit of the team as a whole. If an individual is aware of how their behaviour affects others, such as the activist knowing that reflectors tend to see their behaviour as bullying, then that behaviour can be modified. An example of this in the primary health care setting is to give work that requires a lot of consideration to a reflector, whereas work that needs to be done fast should be given to the activist or pragmatist.

Belbin further developed the role of individuals in teams (Belbin 1981). He analysed performances of business organizations and identified the constituents of successful teams. He found that there were eight different characteristics of individuals that tended to affect how a team worked. Each characteristic had both positive and negative features. Broadly, the groups can be divided into four categories, the leaders (shapers and chairs), the drivers (company workers and finishers), the administrators (team workers and evaluators) and the ideas people (innovators and resource investigators). A team consisting of all four types was generally the most successful. The least successful teams consisted of high achievers, the so called 'Apollo effect'.

*Shapers* tended to be dynamic and impulsive. They needed achievement, were opportunistic rather than conscientious and tended to be tough minded. This ability to lead from the front coupled with their driving force made them ideal project leaders, but they tended to be disruptive in a well balanced team, argumentative and abrasive, becoming impatient and easily frustrated. They tended to clash with other leaders but could form a strong combination with finishers.

*Chair people* were calm, self-confident, trusting, unflappable, with enthusiasm and the ability to communicate with others. These strengths helped guide a team to its objectives, ensuring that each member gave of their best, and these people were particularly good at pulling the team together in a time of crisis. They could, however, be domineering and bossy, intimidating the rest of the team, so that the team became an extension of the chair's ideas. They clashed with shapers over leadership of the group. In a team with both types, only one could be a leader at any one time. They related well with all members of the team.

*Innovators* were independent and imaginative people with a tendency to have original, radical and clever ideas. They produced the vital spark in a team, with the capacity for planning potentially rewarding ideas. They tended, however, to be oversensitive and to become isolated. They related well to the chair and to the team worker and evaluator. Belbin's work suggested they were a key element of a successful team.

*Resource investigators* were communicative and sociable, outgoing and gregarious. They tended to be versatile as well as innovative, but unlike the innovator who created ideas from within, they sought ideas from outside, bringing them to the team. Their strengths showed in the manner in which they sought ideas from outside, brought them back to the team, and integrated them into the ideas of the group thus preventing stagnation. They liked pressure, however, and tended to be complacent without it. They related well with most members of the team, forming a strong combination with shapers and team workers.

*Evaluators* were prudent and hard headed, and tended to be analytic in their approach to problems. They were shrewd judges of situations, keeping interventions to a minimum, hardly ever being wrong. Their great strength was making sure that the team was not making a wrong decision. They had the capacity for thinking through a complex issue, taking all factors into account before giving their opinion. This ability could, however, make them seem aloof and dry. Indeed, they sometimes became boring, over-critical and pessimistic. They related well with the innovator.

*Company worker:* of all team members, Belbin's research showed the company worker to be a key member in a successful business team. They were practical, methodical and hard working, the engine behind any scheme the team might undertake. They were tough minded, yet tolerant, self-controlled and orthodox. They had great organizational flair, turning ideas into manageable projects, clearly defining the tasks that needed to be done. They worked with the team, sacrificing self-interest for the good of the team. These strengths were sometimes weaknesses, so that their singlemindedness could become a lack of flexibility and imagination. They might, too, have difficulty in motivating and inspiring others in the team. They worked well with finishers, shapers and evaluators.

*Team worker:* evaluators monitored the current task; team workers monitored the people in the team. They were sympathetic and sensitive, with a particular interest in how the individuals in the team interacted. They promoted unity in the team, creating a network between team members. They placed group objectives above personal interest, and people before tasks. They were particularly good at coping with awkward people and dealing with disputes. These virtues might, however, lead them to be indecisive at moments of crisis as they preferred to consider all views before acting. They worked well with all team members, but particularly with the organizer and finisher.

*Finisher:* a valuable member of any team, the finisher was painstaking and conscientious, following through tasks to their completion. Although they appeared unflappable, they sometimes suffered internal anxiety due to their need to meet deadlines and targets. They had great capacity for hard work, to the extent that they were sometimes intolerant of slovenly work. The great strength of the finisher was their ability to ensure the team met its obligations, ensuring nothing was overlooked, that the team did not waste time. This obsession with detail could lead to anxiety that might inhibit the team. The finisher worked well with the chair and the evaluator.

These characteristics as described by Belbin are important to consider in maximizing the capacity of the team to function. It is also important to balance a team in other ways, such as the necessary skills to achieve particular tasks. Identifying this skill mix is essential in primary health care as required tasks become more complex, and as skilled personnel become less available. It is estimated that there will be a national shortage of skilled persons by the middle of this decade, with the National Health Service needing to absorb a large part of the school leaver market.

It is vital that a balance is maintained between caring for the

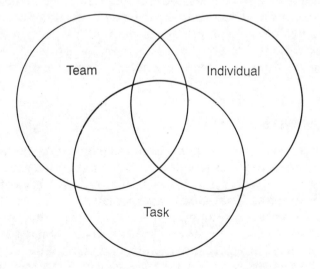

**Fig. 13.1** Key elements to consider in teamwork.

individuals in the group, needs of the team itself and the task in hand. All three need attention and nurturing (see Fig. 13.1). A good 'chair' will be able to develop the team in this way. Likewise, the team worker will see when individuals need particular help. It is essential to complete tasks, but neither individuals nor the team itself should be sacrificed for this end. A cared for team, with members who are valued, will produce quality outcomes and achieve the tasks in hand.

## CHOOSING A TEAM

Industrial teams commonly use psychometric testing such as the Belbin inventory for choosing members. Primary health care teams rarely use these methods, tending to rely on subjective techniques, identifying similarities or even using gut feelings. It is certainly unusual for a general practice team to consider clearly what type of person they are looking for. It is helpful, then, for all members of the team to specifically examine the characteristics needed of the new team member and to identify the criteria against which they would judge applicants. These criteria could include competence in specific clinical skills such as family planning or care of the elderly, and also personal qualities such as the ability to finish a project or meld a team together.

In making overt statements, individuals in the present team avoid the trap of assuming that all are seeking the same particular quality. Given that a good team shows a blend of the characteristics described previously, it can be helpful to assess the current team using these tests, choosing a team member to complement rather than be similar to existing members. Psychometric testing requires the assistance of a trained administrator. An advantage of all this initial preparation is to clarify expectations and structure the interview process, take into account the needs of the team as a whole, and eliminate interviewer bias.

## PROBLEMS WITH TEAMS

Janis describes a common team problem as being 'group-think' (Janis 1982). This occurs when groups become too cohesive and group goals become individual goals. The original task becomes subservient to the needs of the group and individuals to perpetuate their organization. In group-think, the negative implications of risks are not considered. There is a failure to see the ethical or moral implications of a policy. Group members who begin to doubt the group's aims or behaviour are suppressed. Members rarely discuss the business of the team outside itself, and carefully screen out opinions that diverge from those of the group so that unanimity is always reached. They incorrectly reason away material from outside which runs counter to their beliefs and tend to stereotype other teams as being unsuccessful and deviant in some way.

Group-think can be prevented by having a good skill, personality and role mix in the team, coupled with an atmosphere of constructive criticism. Regular evaluation from outside the team is also a powerful protection against group-think. In primary care such external comment is still not common practice.

Other problems can arise from a member's personal agenda becoming more important than the agenda of the group itself. The individual's goals outweigh the task and the team as a whole. A member may, for example, disrupt team cohesion by forming a strong alliance with another member of the team. It should be noted that this may take many forms, for example competition amongst team members or beliefs regarding the achievement of targets. Collusion may also affect the function of a team, as for example when one member of the team conceals another's errors.

Careful selection of the team, clear goals and a common purpose together with honesty and trust, all lead to the development of a strong team. This can only enhance the quality of care offered to the patients.

## FURTHER READING

Bales R.F. (1950) *Interaction Process Analysis. A Method for the Study of Small Groups.* University of Chicago Press, Chicago.

Belbin, M. (1981) *Management Teams.* Heinemann, London.

Honey P. & Mumford A. (1982) *Manual of Learning Styles.* Honey, Maidenhead.

Janis I. (1982) *Groupthink.* Houghton-Mifflin, Boston.

Lewin K. (1948) *Resolving Social Conflicts.* Harper & Row, New York.

Schutz W. (1958) *The Interpersonal Underworld.* Consulting Psychologists Press, Palo Alto.

# Chapter 14

# Medical Audit

Medical audit is a process of measuring the quality of care provided in our practices. The main aim of audit is to improve the standard of care received by our patients. Therefore, before an audit is done, we must consider the nature of quality in general practice.

At the end of this chapter you should:

1 Be aware of the meaning of audit.
2 Understand the process of audit.
3 Have considered the concepts related to quality of care in practice.

## THE AUDIT PROCESS

'The purpose of audit is to identify opportunities and implement improvements in the quality of medical care' (Shaw 1989).

Audit can be viewed as a cycle: standards are set, activity is recorded, comparison between activities and the standard is made, and areas of change are identified to meet the standards. The audit cycle is illustrated in Figure 14.1.

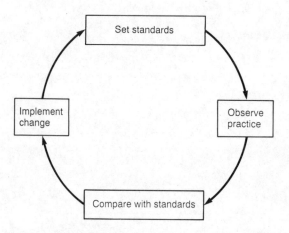

**Fig. 14.1** The audit cycle.

To begin the process of the audit cycle, we must first clarify the definition of a standard and of a criterion. A *criterion* may be defined as an element of care that can be measured in order to assess quality. For example, blood pressure should be measured in all 35–60 year olds every 5 years. A *standard* is the precise count or quality of a criterion that specifies a minimum acceptable level of care. An example of a standard here is that blood pressure shall be recorded in 80% of all 35–60 year olds every 5 years. This shows that it is possible to measure whether or not a particular standard has been met. If it has not been met, then members of the practice can decide what corrective action needs to be taken.

Three main aspects of care are measured under the audit process.

1  *Structure:* 'what do we have and how do we organize it?'; features of an organization that may have an effect on care including buildings, record keeping, staff experience and training.
2  *Process:* 'how we are doing what we do?'; it can be applied to such areas as the medical competence of the clinicians, attitudes of clinicians and other staff to patients, and the teamwork approach to care.
3  *Outcome:* 'are we achieving what we set out to achieve?' The practice should focus on:
   (a)  effectiveness – 'the probability of benefit from a technology or service under normal conditions of use' (Shaw 1989);
   (b)  efficiency – the best possible use of resources; and
   (c)  patient satisfaction – how patients feel about their treatment. This is a difficult area to evaluate, as patients may be satisfied even though they have not been cured, or *vice versa*.

Some examples of broad areas that can be audited are outlined in Table 14.1 (Richards 1991). The measurement of quality is in essence what audit is about. It is clearly important to look at what is meant by quality of care.

We all know quality when we see it: a Rembrandt is clearly of higher quality than any picture drawn by the average person. A Rolls Royce is of higher quality than a Mini; but is a Morris 1000 of higher quality than the Mini, or is a Lamborghini of higher quality than the Rolls?

In commercial settings firms now talk about quality in terms of the concept of zero defect, accepting nothing but the best and not tolerating any deficiency. We would not be satisfied with an airline that advertized that 80% of flights reached their destination. Applying this notion to health care, should we be satisfied that 80% of hypertensives are assessed every year? Clearly there are aspects of medical care in which quality can be quantified, particularly in terms of the outcome of that care.

**Table 14.1**   Examples of Audit Activities.

*Practice activity analysis*
Collecting data prospectively and then pooling and analysing them to compare individual performances, e.g. how long do patients have to wait to see the doctor.

*Case analysis*
Retrospective examination of management in a sample of cases, e.g. review of management of a certain number of cases of carcinoma of the colon to study presentation – diagnosis delay.

*Disease audit*
Assessment of performance for disease management against agreed criteria, e.g. identifying the number of diabetics whose fundi have been examined during the past year.

*Consumer surveys*
Using patients' views about aspects of care, e.g. assessing whether a non-appointment surgery is meeting patients' needs.

*Use of routinely available information*
Analysis of data essential to the running of the practice, e.g. a detailed analysis of PACT data to look at prescribing habits.

*Practice annual reports*
Their use for audit has been limited, but their future role is likely to be extensive.

*Critical incident analysis*
Regular reviews of selected activities in which an error can be shown to have occurred, e.g. a visit not logged, the reasons behind the event, and remedial action to make sure it does not happen again.

Care and quality are internal aspects of the same thing. A person who sees quality and feels it as he works is a person who cares (Pirsig 1974). A person who cares about what he sees and does is bound to have some characteristics of quality.

What is the essence of quality? What features of a service should we look at to decide whether it is quality service? The following seven items may be considered in this context:

1   *Access:* the ability to receive care when you want it. This would include not only waiting times and waiting lists, but also geographical considerations like branch surgeries and physical aspects like access to buildings.
2   *Equity:* providing care without discrimination. This would include perhaps unpopular patients, the last on the surgery list, or the parent who decides against immunization.
3   *Effectiveness:* have the benefits or outcomes which were intended

and desired been achieved? Has the antibiotic cured the illness? This questions the definitions of health and illness.

4  *Acceptability:* is the service acceptable to the user? This would include, for example, administrative procedures, the surgery environment, attitude of the team, and information provided both of the practice and of clinical care.
5  *Efficiency:* have the outcomes been achieved in the best possible way. This includes financial considerations but goes further to include concepts such as skill mix. Costing quality of care is difficult. Consider a patient who has a hernia. Would it be cheaper to improve the turnover of the hospital by getting him earlier, with the reduction of social services costs and other hidden costs to society?
6  *Appropriateness:* examples of dilemmas here would be whether to treat hypertension in the elderly, give antibiotics to children with sore throats, or to children with upper respiratory tract infections and wheeze. In management terms, an example might be whether to add patients to the list while a surgery is running, or whether to ask them to wait until the surgery ends.
7  *Timeliness:* this has always been considered in general practice, such as the idea of deciding when is the optimum time to intervene, whether clinically or administratively. A similar problem applies to hospitals and their waiting lists.

Quality must be a feature of the whole organization, not just of one part. It needs to be integrated as part of the philosophy of the team. In terms of quality issues, each member of the team is as important as another. Each should be recognized for their contributions to the overall quality of the practice.

## AUDIT

Having looked at some of the ideas underlying quality, we can now turn to audit itself – the measure of quality.

Medical audit has been defined by the Department of Health (1990) as:

A frank discussion by doctors on a regular basis without fear of criticism, of the quality of care provided as judged against agreed standards but in a context which allows evolutionary change in such standards.

It is clear from this that audit as perceived by the Department of Health has a strong educational basis for the medical profession. It is important to distinguish between audit for contractual purposes (for contract requirements) and audit for educational purposes (for personal, practice and patient gain). It is also important to note that audit can go further and question the clinical practice of other staff (clinical staff) and the whole service provided.

The audit cycle is shown in Figure 14.1. In practice this involves five steps:

1 Peer review.
2 Setting standards.
3 Reviewing current practice.
4 Deciding on remedial action.
5 Taking action.

*Peer review:* The essence of audit is peer review. This involves being prepared to allow personal professional methods and practice to be scrutinized by colleagues. By comparing clinical practices, norms and standards can be set.

*Setting standards:* As said previously, peer review can help set standards. Standards can also be set by a consensus view within the practice team. Literature reviews and research also help identify appropriate standards.

*Reviewing current practice:* Having decided and set a standard, data have to be collected on current activity. Data collection is a routine task and thought will be given as to who is the appropriate person to undertake this. Computerization has made data manipulation easier, but even greater consideration has to be given to deciding whether or not the data need to be collected and are useful.

*Deciding on remedial action:* Having obtained the data, the team then needs to compare them with the standards set. For example, in an audit of diabetes, the standard set was that all fundi should have been examined within the past 12 months. If there is a 50% success rate, one course of action would be to call back all those who had missed examination either by a separate appointment or by tagging their notes. Another course of action would be to identify why half had been missed. This may result in further education.

*Taking action:* Having decided on the action, it is vital to see that it is actually carried out. It may be that a person in the team needs to be assigned the specific role of ensuring that the action is carried out.

It might be that there is a mismatch between activity and standards. This may be because the standards have been set too high or are unrealistic. Targets which cannot be achieved are of no value. For example, the target of having 100% cervical smears is clearly unrealistic as some women have had hysterectomies and therefore smears are not possible. It must be possible to reach the target or the failure acts as a de-motivator. One aim of audit is to motivate and encourage people towards providing better care.

All general practitioners have to show they are carrying out audits by 1 April 1992. To help general practitioners, the government has set up Medical Audit Advisory Committees (MAAGs) in each region. The main responsibility of the MAAG is to find out whether or not every general practitioner is involved in medical audit. 'MAAGs will be accountable to the FHSA for the institution of regular and systematic medical audit in which all GPs take part. The objective is the participation of all practices by April 1992' (*Health Circular* HC(90) 15).

## CONCLUSION

Audit is a useful process in identifying areas that enable practitioners to provide the best possible care to their patients. It enables all team members to contribute to the efficient and effective provision of care.

## FURTHER READING

Department of Health (1990) *The Quality of Medical Care*. HMSO, London.
Department of Health. *Health Circular* (HC(90) 15).
Irvine D. (1990) *Managing for Quality in General Practice*. King's Fund Centre, London.
Pirsig R.M. (1974) *Zen and the Art of Motorcycle Maintenance*. Corgi Books.
Richards C. (1991) Impact of medical audit advisory groups. *British Medical Journal* **302**, 153–155.
Shaw C. (1989) *Medical Audit. A Hospital Handbook*. Kings Fund Centre, London.

# Chapter 15

# How to Survive the Future

The last few years in general practice have seen more change than ever before and there is a sense for many practices of being on a rollercoaster which is running away, one knows not where. In this climate it is vital for all the members of the practice to feel reasonably comfortable with change and, most importantly, have control of their own destiny. The fulcrum around which this change takes place and the one responsible for making sure that things stay in control is the practice manager. There is no doubt that any but the very smallest practices will need to have a properly trained and effective manager if everyone is to survive and, what's more, enjoy it!

In this book, particularly in the chapter on management, the authors have tried to focus on giving the reader strategies for managing change. Such skills as delegation, motivation, conflict management and forcefield analysis are all vital to this process. Learning these skills and applying them will help considerably to reduce the internal stress and pressures within the practice. However, many of these responses are reactive and ultimately the fate of the practice will depend on a proactive outlook. This means anticipating changes and developments in general practice and planning strategies to cope with them *before* they come about and not after being overtaken by events.

The response of the medical profession to the 1990 contract developments was a classic example of this lack of forethought. Throughout the 1980s a whole series of government discussion papers and policy documents clearly indicated where the thinking at a national level was going. Those general practitioners who read (and understood!) those documents had the opportunity to begin to think about consumer orientation, audit and the achievement of targets long before these were imposed by a government tired of procrastination amongst the medico politicians who continually tried to maintain the *status quo*. As long as 10 years previously those with foresight were warning the profession that if it didn't take responsibility for regulating its own standards then they would be imposed from without and, indeed, that is exactly what happened.

So if one is to survive then it is important to look into the future and see what can be forecast. This can be an exciting exercise and all practices should try it from time to time. It will, of course, be important to take these issues into account when planning the practice's 1 and 5-year plans, as suggested in Chapter 12.

Since the 1990 contract and budget holding developments occurred there has been a major strategy document published by the government (September 1991). *The Health of the Nation* contains quite specific suggestions as to where primary care might be in 10 to 15 years time. The emphasis of this document is on preventive care and the attainment of health care targets in terms of reduction of coronary heart disease, smoking, etc., in the population. There is no doubt that resources and encouragement will be given to practices to follow these philosophies and such activities as the health promotion clinics of the 1990 contract are the first stages in this direction.

Another area where major changes can be expected is within the area of administration of primary care resources. As from 1 April 1991 Regional Health Authorities were responsible for administering the budgets of primary care while knowing very little about the issues of general practice. They will have to learn and it is vital that influential people from within the primary health care team make their voices heard. The Family Health Service Authorities (FHSAs) are in a new role and trying to expand it. Already they are no longer recognizable as the rather amateurish and friendly Family Practitioner Committees (FPCs) of yesteryear.

Many FHSA managers are looking to expand their sphere of influence and are being encouraged by the political climate to encourage new initiatives in primary care. These include applying budget holding principles to other areas besides those already covered by GP fund holding, such as staff training budgets within the practice.

The District Health Authorities are fighting for their existence and it is quite likely that they will be absorbed into a new Primary Care Authority which has responsibilities with regard to hospital services, reacting to the needs of the community. In different parts of the country the scenario may be slightly different but the general trend is recognizable. The consequences of these changes in a few years might well be that there is a single authority overseeing primary care and hospital services and that within this framework GPs will hold their own budgets for the complete administration of their practice and patient services.

This is an exciting scenario and puts general practice in a central position controlling its own destiny. It can be seen that if this were the case then practice managers would need budgeting and accounting skills as a prerequisite for doing the job. If practice managers take over more of this central management role then other members of the staff will have to be trained to take over some of the manager's more traditional roles.

This emphasizes the fact that more and more training is going to be required in this decade for all staff from GP principals to receptionists. The practice manager will be responsible for organizing this training and seeing that it is appropriate for the needs of the learners (Chapter 11). Much of the training may take place within the practice and the manager may have to acquire educational skills to obtain the maximum benefit from these responsibilities.

The 1990s are proving to be a time of great change nationally and internationally, and a recommended read for managers is Charles Handy's *Age of Unreason*. It looks at the whole area of work in the future: how the current expected lifetime working hours are likely to be cut by half and what this will mean to the pattern of our lives; how and where we may work; and what kind of qualifications and experiences we shall need.

With the reduction in the number of younger people entering the workforce, this will lead to difficulties in recruitment for general practice staff in the future. It may be that more sophisticated information technology will be used to enable medical secretaries to work from home, linked by a modem to the surgery. Perhaps all medical records will be computerized. Home working for some people could cut down the cost of the employer, for instance on overheads; space, lighting, heating and furniture. For employees, those tied to home, such as mothers, who have difficulty in finding suitable child care, could work at times to fit in with family commitments.

The demands of the job of a practice manager, whilst varied, interesting and challenging, can be stressful. The constant changes occurring within general practice require great stamina and the ability to respond positively when the team may be in a state of storming (an inevitable response to unwelcome changes). It is essential that managers take sensible steps to survive these challenges.

## SHARING YOUR PROBLEMS

The position of practice manager can be very isolating. Usually there is only one in the practice by the very nature of the job, whereas receptionists, secretaries and nurses often work in teams. The burden of non-clinical management can sometimes feel a heavy one. The stress of these responsibilities can be lightened by meeting with colleagues in similar positions, and the sharing of problems and ideas.

A 'managers only' group enables the free discussion of difficulties associated with managing staff, which are often one of the most complicated areas to cope with. These meetings can range from small, informal gatherings of two or three colleagues, to larger, more organized affairs. The AHCPA has branches throughout the nation, all organized to respond to local needs. If there is not a group in your area, why not start one up? Financial and organizational help is provided and the address of the AHCPA is at the end of Chapter 11.

As can be seen from the above comments there is no question of the practice manager becoming redundant. It is likely that this position will become one of the most important and challenging within the health service as the turn of the century approaches. The challenges can be both exciting and daunting and the intention of this book has been to give practice managers the opportunity to think about, and prepare for, this new and developing role. The authors hope they have been successful in doing this for the reader.

## FURTHER READING

Handy C. (1987) *The Age of Unreason*. Business Books Ltd.
Toffler A. (1970) *Future Shock*. Bodley Head.

# Index

A4 folder
  storage of medical notes, 43–4
accountants
  working with, 65
accounting
  and computerization, 49–50
accounts
  year end, 60, 62, 65
acute prescribing
  and computerization, 49, 55
Adair, John
  and time management, 112
  framework for problem solving, 14
  leadership series of books, 10, 12
  planning cycle model, 13
advertising a job vacancy, 70–71
  for GP trainee, 93
age/sex register, 44
  and computerization, 55
  and GP training, 89
annual report, 6–7, 16, 19
  and computerization, 49–50
  and information of training for office staff,
    25
  and medical audit, 124
answer machines, 80
answering services, 82–3
anti-discrimination legislation, 77
appointment of GP trainee, 93
appointments systems, 41–2
appraisal, 15–16
  and training needs, 97
Association of Health Centre and Practice
    Administrators [AHCPA], 5
  cash flow forecasting sheet, 63–4
  model employment contract, 72
  survey of [1991], 7, 9
  training courses, 99–100
Association of Medical Secretaries, 5
Association of Medical Secretaries, Practice
    Administrators and Receptionists
    [AMSPAR], 5
  training courses, 25, 98, 100
Asthma Training Centre, Stratford, 98
audit, 125–6
  cycle, 15, 122
  examples of activities, 124
  process, 122–5

'trail', 49
  see also medical audit
auditing, 50

Bales' study of group function, 115
banks
  working with, 65–6
Belbin
  analysis of business organization
    performance, 117–19
  inventory, 120
Beveridge, William, 2
Binder Hamlyn Report 1982, 6
bookkeeping, 58–61
briefing people, 13
British Medical Association
  and NHS Act, 2
  and pay and conditions of service in 1960s, 3
  model employment contract, 72
business development loans, 66
business management courses, 99
business plans, 7, 12–13
  and policy making, 11

call forwarding, 81
capital accounts, 63
capitation fees, 2, 4
  for under fives, 27
car allowance for GP trainees, 22, 93
career structure for GPs, 3
Cartwright, Ann
  survey 1967, 4
Cartwright and Anderson Report 1981, 4
case analysis, 124
cash books, 59
cash flow accountancy packages, 50
cash flow forecasting, 50, 63–4
Certificate in Management Studies, 100
cervical cytology
  item of service fee, 4
  and Practice Nurse, 23
changing doctor, 19
  and GP contract 1990, 6
children
  and waiting areas, 40
cleaning of practice premises, 38–9
clinical waste bags, 38